AF669959

Microsurgical Brain Aneurysms

Hans-Jakob Steiger • Nima Etminan
Daniel Hänggi

Microsurgical Brain Aneurysms

Illustrated Concepts and Cases

Springer

Hans-Jakob Steiger
Neurochirurgische Klinik
Universitätsklinikum Düsseldorf
Düsseldorf
Germany

Daniel Hänggi
Neurochirurgische Klinik
Universitätsklinikum Düsseldorf
Düsseldorf
Germany

Nima Etminan
Neurochirurgische Klinik
Universitätsklinikum Düsseldorf
Düsseldorf
Germany

Medical Artwork by Christine Opfermann-Rüngeler, Düsseldorf

ISBN 978-3-662-45678-1 ISBN 978-3-662-45679-8 (eBook)
DOI 10.1007/978-3-662-45679-8
Springer Heidelberg New York Dordrecht London

Library of Congress Control Number: 2014960135

© Springer-Verlag Berlin Heidelberg 2015
This work is subject to copyright. All rights are reserved by the Publisher, whether the whole or part of the material is concerned, specifically the rights of translation, reprinting, reuse of illustrations, recitation, broadcasting, reproduction on microfilms or in any other physical way, and transmission or information storage and retrieval, electronic adaptation, computer software, or by similar or dissimilar methodology now known or hereafter developed. Exempted from this legal reservation are brief excerpts in connection with reviews or scholarly analysis or material supplied specifically for the purpose of being entered and executed on a computer system, for exclusive use by the purchaser of the work. Duplication of this publication or parts thereof is permitted only under the provisions of the Copyright Law of the Publisher's location, in its current version, and permission for use must always be obtained from Springer. Permissions for use may be obtained through RightsLink at the Copyright Clearance Center. Violations are liable to prosecution under the respective Copyright Law.
The use of general descriptive names, registered names, trademarks, service marks, etc. in this publication does not imply, even in the absence of a specific statement, that such names are exempt from the relevant protective laws and regulations and therefore free for general use.
While the advice and information in this book are believed to be true and accurate at the date of publication, neither the authors nor the editors nor the publisher can accept any legal responsibility for any errors or omissions that may be made. The publisher makes no warranty, express or implied, with respect to the material contained herein.

Printed on acid-free paper

Springer is part of Springer Science+Business Media (www.springer.com)

This book is for the residents and young neurosurgeons deciding to embark upon vascular neurosurgery, which is a life-long journey with an uncertain destination.

Preface

Microsurgery of cerebral aneurysms has gone a long way since the publication of the first book on the topic by Walter Dandy in 1944. Development of aneurysm surgery coincided to a large degree with the development of microsurgical techniques in general. Accumulation of detailed technical knowledge and also pathophysiological understanding led to the publication of a monumental three-volume text by John Fox in 1983. Aneurysm microsurgery was special, it was difficult, and it was not for everyone. It was challenging. The advent of endovascular coiling in 1990 had a deep impact on the microsurgical landscape. It was realized long before the publication of the ISAT results (International Subarachnoid Aneurysm Trial) in 2002 that the endovascular approach could treat aneurysms of the basilar apex with much less risk than microsurgery. Publication of the ISAT results involved a number of consequences. Microsurgery has become the second choice for cases in which the endovascular therapist encounters difficulties. Depending on the local team, more difficult aneurysms could be left for surgery. On the other hand, the neurosurgeon does not need to operate on all difficult aneurysms. Surgery can avoid risky cases. The team interaction is certainly critical for the balance between the two disciplines. There are currently large differences across Europe with regard to the proportion of aneurysms being coiled and clipped. These differences are essentially a consequence of the competitive nature of coiling and clipping. To eliminate factors of competition among disciplines, the neurovascular surgeon competent with microsurgical and endovascular techniques emerged in the United States and Japan, among others. In Europe, attempts were made to establish such a system in a few places but without much success. Therefore, the interdisciplinary team approach remains the European standard. The current average relation between clipping and coiling is quite balanced (around half and half) in Europe.

Aneurysm microsurgery remains special and challenging. Microsurgical techniques are innate to the current generation of neurosurgeons. As such, a modern book of aneurysm microsurgery can avoid repeating basic microsurgical techniques. This was the basis when we decided to analyze our experience of the last decades and summarize essential clues for success.

Technical development of aneurysm microsurgery was largely stunned by the advent of endovascular therapy. Since it is becoming quite clear that microsurgical techniques for brain aneurysms will be needed at least for the next decades, we are convinced that technical development must be intensified.

At our center, the traditional large openings resulting in stigmatizing disfigurations have been replaced by small targeted craniotomies. It is a main focus of the present book to introduce the targeted approaches and the resulting specific clipping techniques.

Management of subarachnoid hemorrhage and the technical act of clipping a brain aneurysm requires a deeper understanding of pathophysiology and hemodynamics because these factors determine the typical constellations, configuration, and consequently approach and clipping techniques. Therefore, the hemodynamic principles and resulting types of aneurysm are depicted in the first part of this book.

Düsseldorf, Germany
July, 2014

Hans-Jakob Steiger
Nima Etminan
Daniel Hänggi

Contents

Abbreviations

A1	Precommunicating segment of anterior cerebral artery
A2	Postcommunicating segment of anterior cerebral artery
ACA	Anterior cerebral artery
AChA	Anterior choroidal artery
Acom	Anterior communicating artery
AICA	Anterior inferior cerebellar artery
AVM	Arteriovenous malformation
BA	Basilar artery
CCT	Cranial computed tomography
CIRS	Critical incident reporting systems
CSF	Cerebrospinal fluid
DSA	Digital subtraction angiography
EC-IC	Extracranial to intracranial
EVD	External ventricular drainage
HHU	Heinrich Heine University, Düsseldorf
ICA	Internal carotid artery
ICG	Indocyanine green
ICP	Intracranial pressure
ICU	Intensive care unit
M&M	Morbidity and mortality
M1	Proximal segment of middle cerebral artery
M2	Main branches of middle cerebral artery
MAP	Mean arterial pressure
MCA	Middle cerebral artery
MTT	Mean transit time
OR	Operating room
PCA	Posterior cerebral artery
Pcom	Posterior communicating artery
pCT	Perfusion CT
PICA	Posterior inferior cerebellar artery
SAH	Subarachnoid hemorrhage
SCA	Superior cerebellar artery
STA	Superficial temporal artery
TCD	Transcranial Doppler
VA	Vertebral artery
WFNS	World Federation of Neurosurgical Societies

1 The Current State of Aneurysm Microsurgery

The two burning questions regarding the management of cerebral aneurysms currently concern whether to use clip or coil and what to do with incidental aneurysms. Further issues that require continuing attention and research are primary and secondary damage following subarachnoid hemorrhage (i.e., delayed cerebral ischemia) and perhaps primary prevention of cerebral aneurysm formation by pharmaceutical treatment.

1.1 Clip or Coil?

Microsurgical treatment has become a second-choice method of care for intracranial aneurysms that appear to be not easily amenable to endovascular therapy [1]. A neurosurgical service not providing both treatment modalities can no longer offer competent care of patients with ruptured or unruptured aneurysms.

In many clinical situations, there is insufficient evidence for a clear decision with regard to the optimum mode of treatment. There is usually a gray zone where arguments for both options can be found. It is therefore an accepted requirement that the neurosurgeon and the endovascular therapist decide together on the basis of the patient's clinical condition, the configuration of the aneurysm as shown on digital subtraction angiography and CT or MR angiography, and their personal experience. Location is an important factor for the decision. Aneurysms of the basilar artery are clearly the domain of endovascular management, for which neurosurgical services do not have the necessary proficiency, but peripheral aneurysms of all vascular territories are still the domain of microsurgery in many centers. Aneurysms of the main bifurcation of the middle cerebral artery (MCA) are within a gray zone, for which there are arguments and data favoring either treatment modality.

Aneurysm size and neck configuration should not play a significant role in the treatment decision. Larger aneurysms and broad-based aneurysms are more difficult for both endovascular and microsurgical techniques, whereas small or

H.-J. Steiger et al., *Microsurgical Brain Aneurysms: Illustrated Concepts and Cases*,
DOI 10.1007/978-3-662-45679-8_1, © Springer-Verlag Berlin Heidelberg 2015

narrow-necked aneurysms are simpler and safer to treat with both methods.

It would not be realistic to negate treatment logistics in choosing the treatment modality. If the experience of the available endovascular or microsurgical partner clearly dominates, this factor should be considered.

A more difficult question is the value of the patient's wishes in the situation of acute subarachnoid hemorrhage. Patients are often cognitively impaired after acute subarachnoid hemorrhage, and they have limited access to scientific knowledge and to second opinions, because treatment decisions must be made under time pressure. Last but not least, the process of informing the patient must be done cautiously, without causing additional stress, in order not to provoke aneurysm rerupture. In the situation of subarachnoid hemorrhage, therefore, the therapists usually decide on the treatment modality, taking account of any preferences clearly stated by the patient. After the decision, the recommendation is transmitted to the patient with a degree of detailed information appropriate to his or her condition.

1.2 To Treat or Not to Treat Incidental Aneurysms?

The principal treatment indication is rarely in question with ruptured aneurysms, apart from some World Federation of Neurosurgical Societies (WFNS) grade 5 hemorrhages with severe early brain injury and uncontrollable intracranial pressure [2]. In view of the high prevalence of unruptured intracranial aneurysms (UIAs) in the general population (2–3 %) and the fact that only a fraction of these rupture during the lifetime of the individual harboring the UIA, the appropriate assessment of an indication for treatment of an incidental aneurysm is somewhat more challenging [3]. A number of studies give us some estimate of the natural history of incidental aneurysms, the specific risk factors for aneurysm rupture, and the risk of morbidity and mortality associated with treatment [4–8]. However, most studies on the natural history of UIAs have been partially biased through specific selection of subgroups, so that controversy continues regarding the true natural history of UIAs [9, 10]. Nevertheless, aneurysm size and location can be considered the major risk factors for rupture of incidental aneurysms. Here, the data from the International Study of Unruptured Intracranial Aneurysms (ISUIA) [8] and the Unruptured Cerebral Aneurysm Study of Japan (UCAS Japan) [7] have generally suggested a low 5-year risk of rupture (1–2 %) for incidental aneurysms with a maximum diameter below 7 mm. Interestingly, the more recent data from the UCAS Japan study [7] suggested distinctly higher rupture risks for aneurysms of the anterior or posterior communicating artery and of lobulated shape, compared with other aneurysms of the anterior circulation and those of nonlobulated morphology. Risk factors of second priority include previous aneurysmal subarachnoid hemorrhage, family history of UIAs or subarachnoid hemorrhage, Japanese or Finnish ethnicity, untreated hypertension, active smoking, and associated collagen diseases.

Although aneurysm size is a major risk factor for rupture, it is also the main risk factor (in addition to patient age) for treatment complications and morbidity. Pooled data from a meta-analysis of surgical and endovascular repair of UIAs suggest an overall 6–7 % risk of permanent morbidity or mortality [6, 11]. In detail, the treatment risks for small aneurysms of the anterior circulation amount to approximately 1 % per mm in diameter for both treatment modalities. The risk of endovascular obliteration in the posterior circulation appeared comparable to the risk for the anterior circulation, but the complications for microsurgery were twice as high in the ISUIA data set: that is, the risk of poor outcome 1 year after microsurgical obliteration amounted to some 50 % for giant posterior circulation aneurysms [8]. Ultimately, the assessment of patients with UIAs should be multifactorial and ideally should weigh the estimated risk of rupture against the risk of treatment in a patient with a UIA (Fig. 1.1). Importantly, this assessment should account for the fact that the lifetime risk of rupture, especially in patients younger than 40 years or in patients with the aforementioned risk factors, may be stochastic and thus difficult to estimate based on the currently available data.

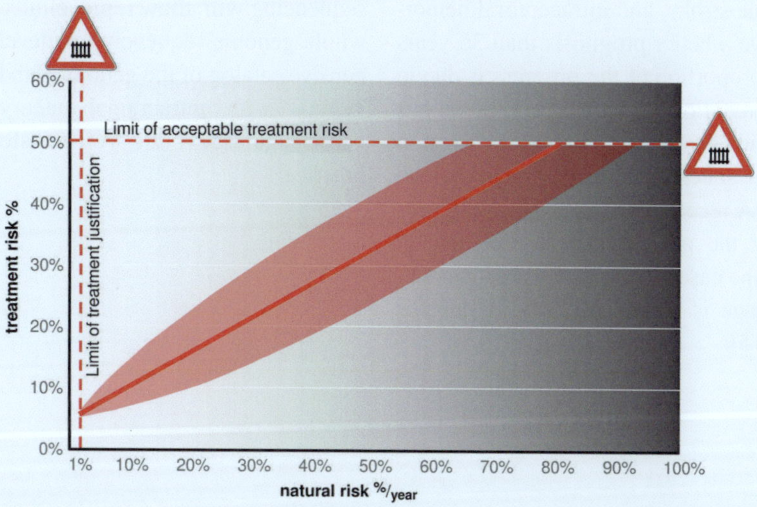

Fig. 1.1 In general, the risk of treatment is related to the natural risk of rupture in a more or less linear way. Therefore, aneurysm size is a questionable argument for treatment. It is our opinion that independently of the exact relation of the estimated risk of treatment and the estimated natural risk of the aneurysms, some absolute boundaries should be respected in view of the uncertainties associated with risk assessment. We would not recommend surgery or endovascular coiling for any aneurysm with an estimated risk of rupture less than 1 % per year, and we would not recommend surgery or endovascular obliteration to any patient in a stable condition if we estimate the odds for an unfavorable outcome to be close to 50–50 or worse

1.3 The Enigma of Secondary Ischemic Damage Following Subarachnoid Hemorrhage

Nimodipine, hypertensive therapy, and monitoring of cerebral perfusion were introduced into clinical practice in the 1980s, and there is no doubt that they have substantially improved outcome. The most apparent progress in the treatment of aneurysmal subarachnoid hemorrhage is reflected in the distinct reduction of mortality [12]. Whereas data from 1980 indicated an overall case fatality rate of about 55 %, extrapolation suggested a decrease to some 30 % around 2010. The reasons for this improvement are not only a consequence of the introduction of nimodipine, hypertensive therapy, and monitoring of cerebral perfusion, however. Patients with traumatic brain injury, ischemic stroke, and intracerebral hemorrhage also have a better prognosis than 30 years ago, so what proportion of the progress is due to better management of the specific complications of subarachnoid hemorrhage and what proportion is due to better general care in the intensive care unit [13, 14]? A recent analysis of our own cases treated during the past decade showed that at least 50 % of the case fatality rate with subarachnoid hemorrhage is related to early or delayed brain injury [15].

1.4 Primary Prevention of Aneurysm Formation

Even as hypertension and smoking are increasingly established risk factors, the genetic factors responsible for familial clustering are still not well enough defined to carry clinical implications. Genome-wide association studies of intracranial aneurysms have the potential to improve our understanding of factors affecting aneurysm growth and rupture. But instead of only one or two genes, multiple loci seem to play a role for aneurysm development and rupture [16, 17]. Furthermore, environmental factors interfere with genetic preponderance, and rupture may be linked to genetic factors other than the formation of aneurysms. Although we are in the midst of a technological revolution in which next-generation sequencing will allow rapid, clinically affordable whole-genome sequencing to develop a comprehensive catalog of the genomic landscape of individuals with intracranial aneurysms, current knowledge does not yet transfer to clinical practice.

References

1. Molyneux AJ, Kerr RS, Birks J, Ramzi N, Yarnold J, Sneade M, et al. Risk of recurrent subarachnoid haemorrhage, death, or dependence and standardised mortality ratios after clipping or coiling of an intracranial aneurysm in the International Subarachnoid Aneurysm Trial (ISAT): long-term follow-up. Lancet Neurol. 2009;8:427–33.
2. Bailes JE, Spetzler RF, Hadley MN, Baldwin HZ. Management morbidity and mortality of poor-grade aneurysm patients. J Neurosurg. 1990;72:559–66.
3. Vernooij MW, Ikram MA, Tanghe HL, Vincent AJ, Hofman A, Krestin GP, et al. Incidental findings on brain MRI in the general population. N Engl J Med. 2007;357:1821–8.
4. Greving JP, Wermer MJ, Brown Jr RD, Morita A, Juvela S, Yonekura M, et al. Development of the PHASES score for prediction of risk of rupture of intracranial aneurysms: a pooled analysis of six prospective cohort studies. Lancet Neurol. 2014;13:59–66.
5. Juvela S, Poussa K, Lehto H, Porras M. Natural history of unruptured intracranial aneurysms: a long-term follow-up study. Stroke. 2013;44:2414–21.
6. Kotowski M, Naggara O, Darsaut TE, Nolet S, Gevry G, Kouznetsov E, et al. Safety and occlusion rates of surgical treatment of unruptured intracranial aneurysms: a systematic review and meta-analysis of the literature from 1990 to 2011. J Neurol Neurosurg Psychiatry. 2013;84:42–8.
7. UCAS Japan Investigators, Morita A, Kirino T, Hashi K, Aoki N, Fukuhara S, et al. The natural course of unruptured cerebral aneurysms in a Japanese cohort. N Engl J Med. 2012;366:2474–82.
8. Wiebers DO, Whisnant JP, Huston 3rd J, Meissner I, Brown Jr RD, Piepgras DG, et al.; International Study of Unruptured Intracranial Aneurysms Investigators. Unruptured intracranial aneurysms: natural history, clinical outcome, and risks of surgical and endovascular treatment. Lancet. 2003;362:103.
9. Brown Jr RD. Controversy: clipping of asymptomatic intracranial aneurysm that is <7 mm: yes or no? Stroke. 2013;44(6 Suppl 1):S96.
10. Steinberg GK. Controversy: clipping of asymptomatic intracranial aneurysm that is <7 mm: yes. Stroke. 2013;44(6 Suppl 1):S97–9.
11. Naggara ON, Lecler A, Oppenheim C, Meder JF, Raymond J. Endovascular treatment of intracranial unruptured aneurysms: a systematic review of the literature on safety with emphasis on subgroup analyses. Radiology. 2012;263:828–35.
12. Lovelock CE, Rinkel GJ, Rothwell PM. Time trends in outcome of subarachnoid hemorrhage: population-based study and systematic review. Neurology. 2010;74:1494–501.
13. Béjot Y, Rouaud O, Durier J, Caillier M, Marie C, Freysz M, et al. Decrease in the stroke case fatality rates in a French population-based twenty-year study. A comparison between men and women. Cerebrovasc Dis. 2007;24:439–44.
14. Biotti D, Jacquin A, Boutarbouch M, Bousquet O, Durier J, Ben Salem D, et al. Trends in case-fatality rates in hospitalized nontraumatic subarachnoid hemorrhage: results of a population-based study in Dijon, France, from 1985 to 2006. Neurosurgery. 2010;66:1039–43.
15. Beseoglu K, Holtkamp K, Steiger HJ, Hänggi D. Fatal aneurysmal subarachnoid haemorrhage: causes of 30-day in-hospital case fatalities in a large single-centre historical patient cohort. Clin Neurol Neurosurg. 2013;115:77–81.
16. Hussain I, Duffis EJ, Gandhi CD, Prestigiacomo CJ. Genome-wide association studies of intracranial aneurysms: an update. Stroke. 2013;44:2670–5.
17. Yasuno K, Bilguvar K, Bijlenga P, Low SK, Krischek B, Auburger G, et al. Genome-wide association study of intracranial aneurysm identifies three new risk loci. Nat Genet. 2010;42:420–5.

2 Pathophysiology and Anatomy

2.1 Terminal Versus Lateral Aneurysms

More than 90 % of all saccular aneurysms arise from bifurcations or appear at the origin of small side branches (percentages are approximate) [1, 2]:

- Middle cerebral artery main bifurcation (15–30 %)
- Anterior communicating artery (20–30 %)
- Internal carotid–posterior communicating artery (15 %)
- Basilar tip (5 %)

  Rare bifurcation aneurysm locations:
- Internal carotid artery bifurcation (2 %)
- Internal carotid–anterior choroidal artery (1–2 %)
- Pericallosal–callosomarginal artery (2 %)
- Basilar–superior cerebellar artery (2 %)
- Vertebral artery–posterior inferior cerebellar artery (2 %)
- Vertebrobasilar junction (1 %)
- Basilar–anterior inferior cerebellar artery (0.5–1 %)

The reported frequency at different sites varies somewhat among different publications and also between series of ruptured and unruptured aneurysms. In particular, aneurysms at the anterior communicating artery are more frequent in series of ruptured aneurysms. In contrast, in pediatric and familial cases, aneurysms appear to occur rarely at the anterior communicating artery.

The distinction between terminal aneurysms and lateral, side branch-related aneurysms is somewhat artificial (Fig. 2.1). In fact, some asymmetry of the bifurcation is common also with terminal aneurysms in that one of the two branches is larger than the other. If the difference in the diameter of the branches is significant, the smaller branch appears as a side branch. The diameters of the side branches also correlate with the angle between the afferent artery and the branches. In case of a large asymmetry between the branches, the larger branch continues more or less in the direction of the afferent artery, while the smaller branch originates more or less at a 90° angle.

H.-J. Steiger et al., *Microsurgical Brain Aneurysms: Illustrated Concepts and Cases*,
DOI 10.1007/978-3-662-45679-8_2, © Springer-Verlag Berlin Heidelberg 2015

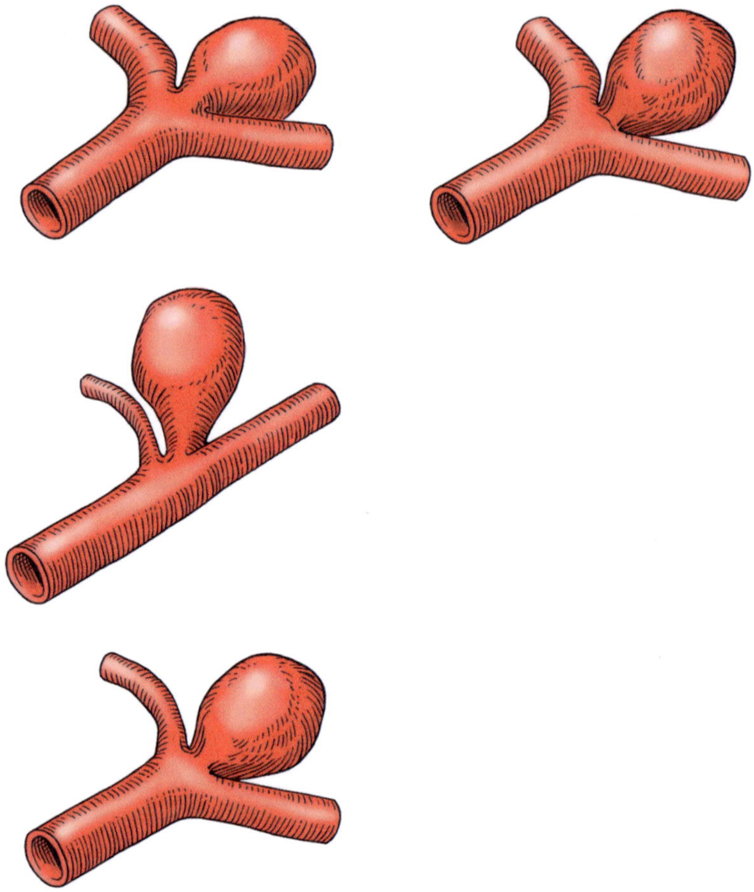

Fig. 2.1 Terminal versus lateral aneurysms. Some asymmetry of the bifurcation or the aneurysm projection is necessary for flow in the aneurysm. If the diameter of the branches differs significantly, the smaller branch appears as a side branch. An aneurysm in relation to a small side branch is called a *lateral aneurysm*, whereas an aneurysm between branches of similar diameter is called a *terminal aneurysm*. The diameters of the side branches also correlate with the angle between the afferent artery and the branches. If there is a large asymmetry between the branches, the larger branch continues more or less in the direction of the afferent artery, and the small branch originates more or less at a 90° angle

2.2 Geometry of Bifurcations

Extracranial arterial bifurcations often show an acute angle between the branches, as in the case of the abdominal aorta, with an acute angle between the common iliac arteries. In contrast, intracranial arteries most often develop a blunt angle between the branches. The reason for this peculiarity is not obvious, but everyday experience confirms this rule. The most logical explanation is that the angle is related to the shape of the arterial environment. If an artery passes through a longitudinal organ such as an extremity, the bifurcations have acute angles, but if arteries pass through an essentially round organ such as the brain, the bifurcations are T-shaped.

In principle, bifurcations of cerebral arteries and the projection of aneurysms could assume any three-dimensional configuration; afferent and efferent arteries need not necessarily lie in a flat plane. In reality, however, there is always a smooth transition from the direction of the afferent vessel to the direction of the branches (Fig. 2.2). Therefore, it is best to imagine the bifurcations as lying on a curved plane.

The diameters of the branches are related, given that the flow velocities in the cerebral arteries vary little. Therefore, in the case of equal branches, the relative diameter of the branches in comparison to the afferent artery corresponds to the square root of 0.5 (i.e., 0.7). If the branches are unequal, the sum of the cross-sectional areas of the branches adds to the cross section of the afferent artery. Figure 2.3 shows some examples of size relations of afferent and efferent arteries.

The intracranial internal carotid artery (ICA) has two typical configurations (Fig. 2.4). The terminal bifurcation regularly assumes the typical T shape, but with variable asymmetry of the diameters of the middle cerebral artery (MCA) and the anterior communicating artery (Acom), the relative size of the posterior communicating artery (Pcom) determines the direction of the distal ICA. The orifice of the Pcom usually is located in the ventral midline of the ICA. In approximately 70 % of individuals, the Pcom is small and constitutes a typical side branch; the distal ICA continues in the direction of the proximal ICA. In about 30 %, however, the Pcom is larger than 2 mm and supplies the posterior cerebral artery, leading to a dorsal deviation of the distal ICA. The diameter of the distal ICA in this situation is also smaller than the diameter of the proximal ICA. The anterior choroidal artery uniformly has a small diameter and is a typical side branch of the ICA.

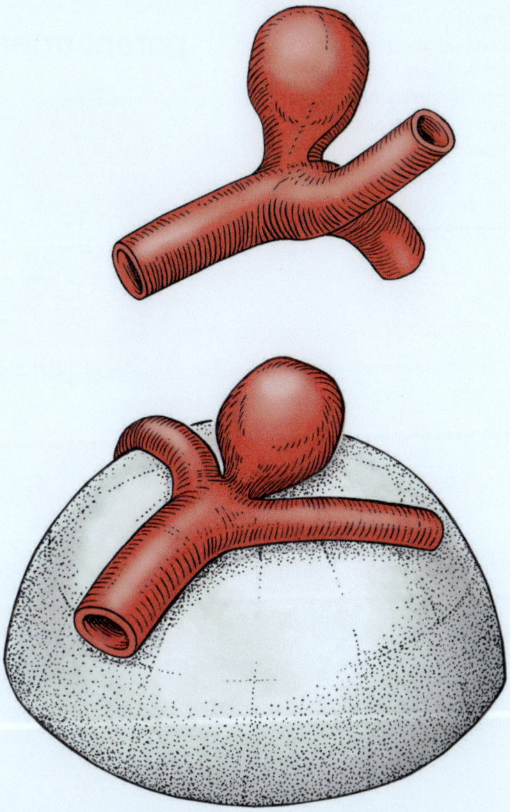

Fig. 2.2 Geometry of bifurcations. Intracranial arterial bifurcations most often have a blunt angle between the branches. In principle, bifurcations of cerebral arteries and the projection of aneurysms could assume any three-dimensional configuration, but in reality, the bifurcations can be imagined as lying on a curved plane. The projection of an aneurysm, however, is not confined to this plane

The anterior cerebral artery bifurcation often displays a few features in patients with aneurysms at the anterior communicating artery (Acom) that differ from the norm (Fig. 2.5). Most often the size of the ACAs in patients with ACA aneurysms is clearly asymmetric. Furthermore, progressive elongation of the ACAs leads to distortion of the ACA, so that

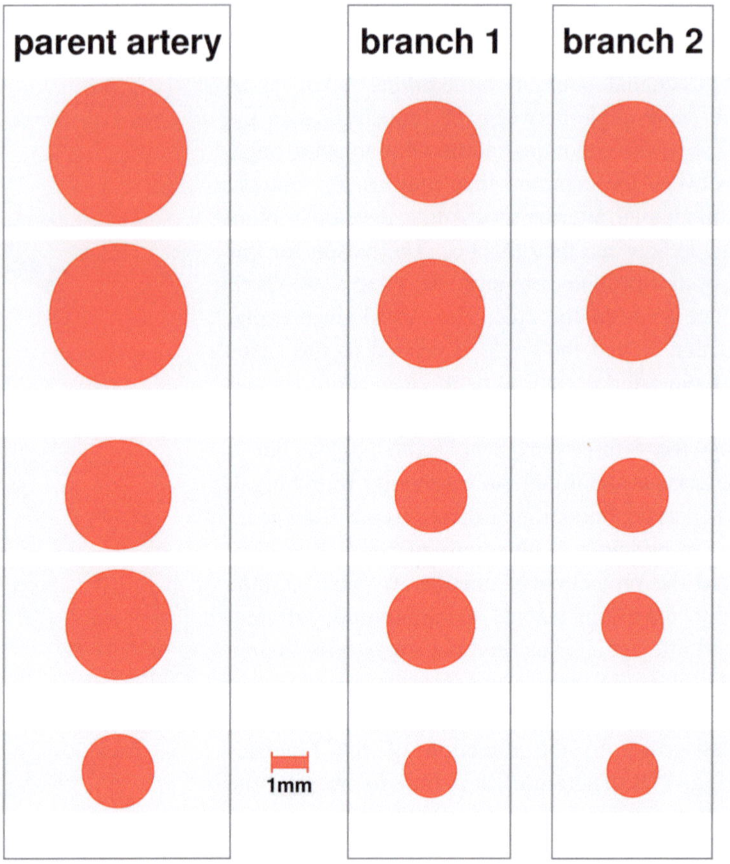

Fig. 2.3 The diameters of cerebral artery branches are related. The area of inflow equals approximately the sum of the areas of the branches. This illustration shows some examples of size relations of afferent and efferent arteries

one A2 segment lies more anteriorly than the other. In about 80 % of these cases, the A2 segment on the side of the dominant A1 lies more posteriorly than the contralateral A2 [3]. With a frontolateral approach to the Acom aneurysm, this predominant configuration (also called the open configuration) allows for easy visualization of the entire Acom complex and particularly both A2 segments. In contrast, in approximately 20 % of patients with an Acom aneurysm, the Acom is turned the other way, so that the A2 on the side of the dominant A1 lies anteriorly. This configuration (also called the closed configuration) is problematic for an anterolateral approach because the contralateral A2 origin hides behind the ipsilateral A2.

A further particular anatomical property of the Acom complex is important. In a small percentage of patients, the A2 divides early into two main trunks, resulting in three A2 segments. If the surgeon is unaware of this special configuration, the risk of inadvertently occluding the third branch with the aneurysm clip becomes significant. On the other hand, an unpaired pericallosal artery (azygos A2) is a constellation associated with aneurysms at the origin of the callosomarginal arteries. On average, the azygos A2 variant is seen in approximately 3 % of angiograms [4].

The MCA bifurcation in aneurysm patients also exhibits some typical features that are relevant for microsurgical treatment. The MCA bifurcation usually is a typical T-shaped bifurcation. A trifurcation is rare. As in the case of the anterior cerebral artery, the M1 segment often has undergone substantial elongation during life, leading to a high-lying and curved course. The

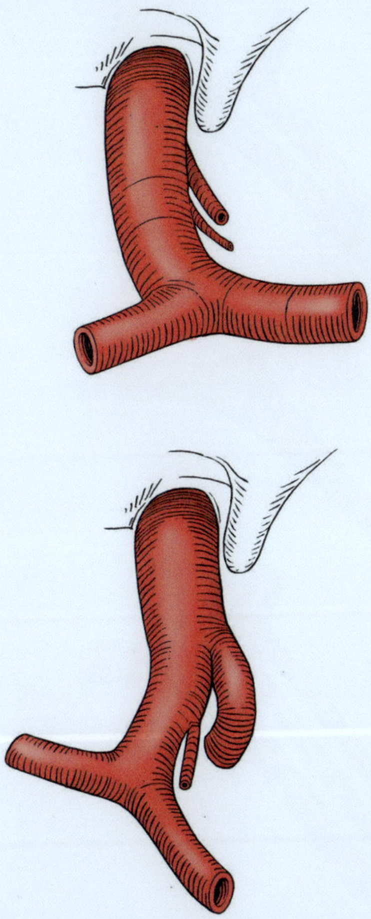

Fig. 2.4 The intracranial internal carotid artery (ICA) has two typical configurations, depending on the size of the posterior communicating artery (Pcom). If the Pcom is small and constitutes a typical side branch, the distal ICA continues in the direction of the proximal ICA. If the Pcom is large and supplies the posterior cerebral artery, the distal ICA turns upward. The anterior choroidal artery uniformly has a small diameter and is a typical side branch of the ICA

distal M1 then actually can lie behind the bifurcation when the MCA bifurcation is approached through the Sylvian fissure (Fig. 2.6). In this situation, we recommend approaching and exposing the distal M1 between the M2 trunks.

Cerebral aneurysms are commonly associated with anomalies of the circle of Willis. The most frequently seen combination is the Acom aneurysm associated with hypoplasia of one anterior cerebral artery. According to various authors, the first segments of the anterior cerebral arteries (A1) are clearly asymmetric in approximately 80 % of patients with an aneurysm at the Acom, whereas the prevalence of unequal A1 segments in healthy individuals is estimated to be only 10–15 % [2, 5, 6]. Furthermore, Acom aneurysms arise consistently at the crotch between the dominant A1 and the communicating artery.

Thrombosis or therapeutic ligation of the internal carotid artery also constitutes a well-known risk factor for subsequent formation of saccular aneurysms [7]. Occlusion of other cerebral arteries has also been associated with an increased incidence of aneurysms of the patent blood channels.

Another category of geometrical variations associated with aneurysms is arteriovenous malformations (AVMs). Between 10 and 30 % of AVM patients are reported to have associated feeder aneurysms [8, 9]. Aneurysms associated with AVMs are located either on the feeder vessels or at common sites of the circle of Willis. The aneurysm-promoting effect of arterial hypoplasia, occlusion, and AVMs is named “hemodynamic stress” [10].

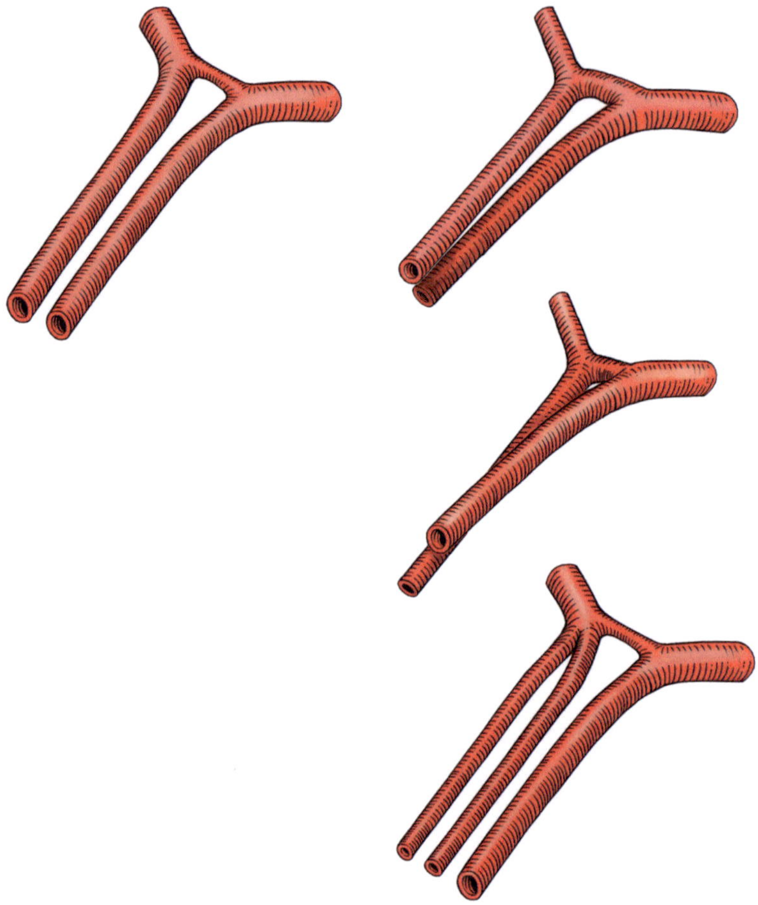

Fig. 2.5 Variations of the anterior communicating artery (Acom) complex. Most often, the size of the A1 segments in patients with ACA aneurysms is clearly asymmetric. Furthermore, progressive elongation of the A1s leads to rotation of the ACA, resulting usually in a more posterior origin of the A2 segment on the side of the dominant A1. The other variant, resulting in a more posterior position of the contralateral A2, is rare. Sometimes, an A2 divides early into two main trunks, resulting in three A2 segments. If the surgeon is unaware of this special configuration, the risk of inadvertently occluding the third branch with the aneurysm clip becomes significant

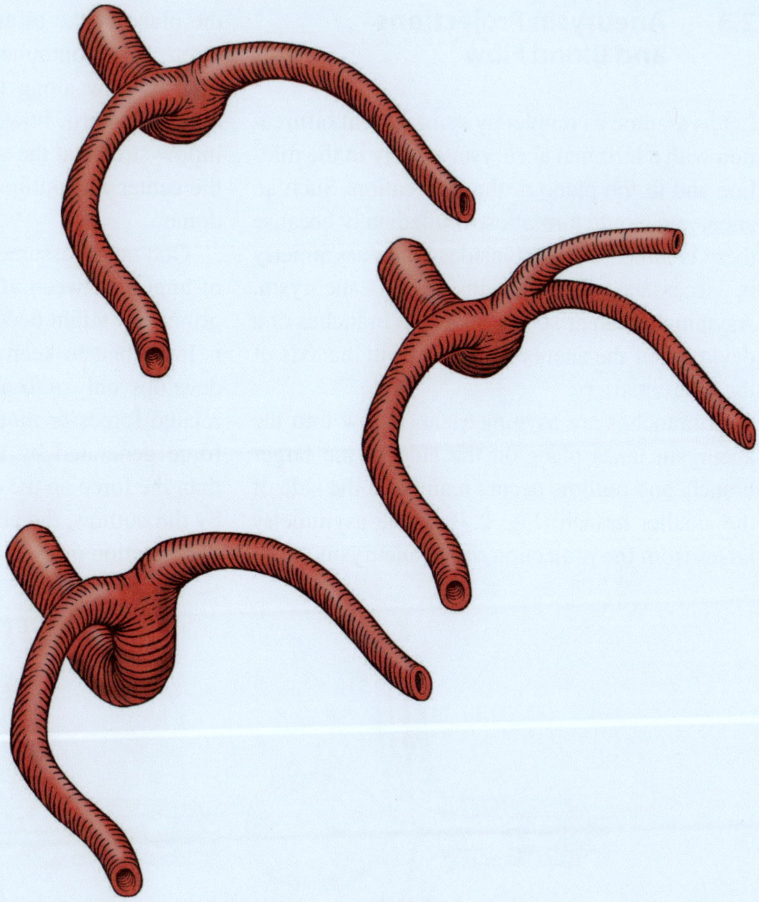

Fig. 2.6 The MCA bifurcation is usually a typical T-shaped bifurcation. A trifurcation is rare. As in the case of the anterior cerebral artery, the M1 segment often has undergone substantial elongation during life, leading to a high-lying and curved course of the M1. The distal M1 then can lie behind the bifurcation if the MCA bifurcation is approached through the Sylvian fissure

2.3 Aneurysm Projections and Blood Flow

Let us assume a completely symmetrical bifurcation with a terminal aneurysm exactly in the midline and in the plane of the bifurcation. Such an aneurysm would thrombose immediately because there is almost no flow inside. Some asymmetry is necessary for flow inside an aneurysm. Asymmetry can arise from unequal branches or a deviation of the aneurysmal axis from the axis of the afferent artery.

If branches are asymmetrical, inflow into the aneurysm takes place on the side of the larger branch, and outflow occurs mainly on the side of the smaller branch (Fig. 2.7). If the asymmetry arises from the projection of the aneurysm out of the plane of the bifurcation, inflow occurs most often as a continuation of the afferent artery, with outflow along the other walls. There is a second pattern, however, with reflection of the inflow stream at the wall of the aneurysm toward the center and outflow along all the walls of the dome.

One might assume that a great many varieties of angles between afferent artery and aneurysm projection might occur, but this is not the case. It is important to keep in mind that the aneurysm develops only into a direction where the flow-related forces or moments are in balance. If the force generated by the inflow stream is larger than the force on the contralateral wall generated by the outflow, the aneurysm will slowly tilt into the direction of the inflow stream.

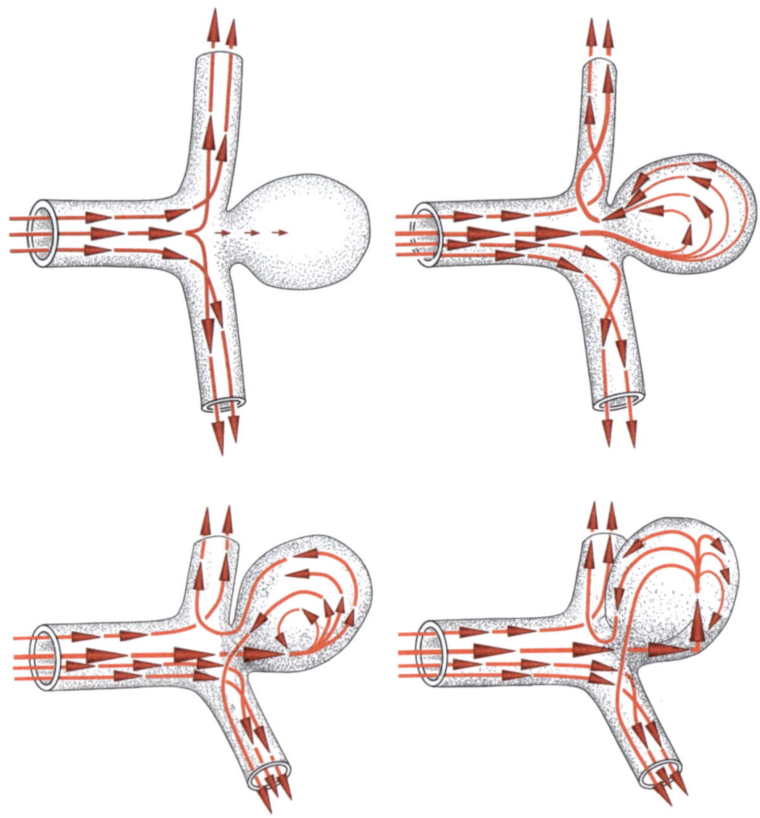

Fig. 2.7 Aneurysm projections and blood flow: Some asymmetry is necessary for flow inside a terminal aneurysm. Asymmetry can arise from unbalanced flow through the branches or from a deviation of the aneurysmal axis from the axis of the afferent artery. Inflow into the aneurysm takes place on the side of the larger branch, with outflow mainly on the side of the smaller branch. If the asymmetry arises from the projection of the aneurysm out of the bifurcation plane, there are two dominant flow patterns in the fundus, depending on the projection of the aneurysm

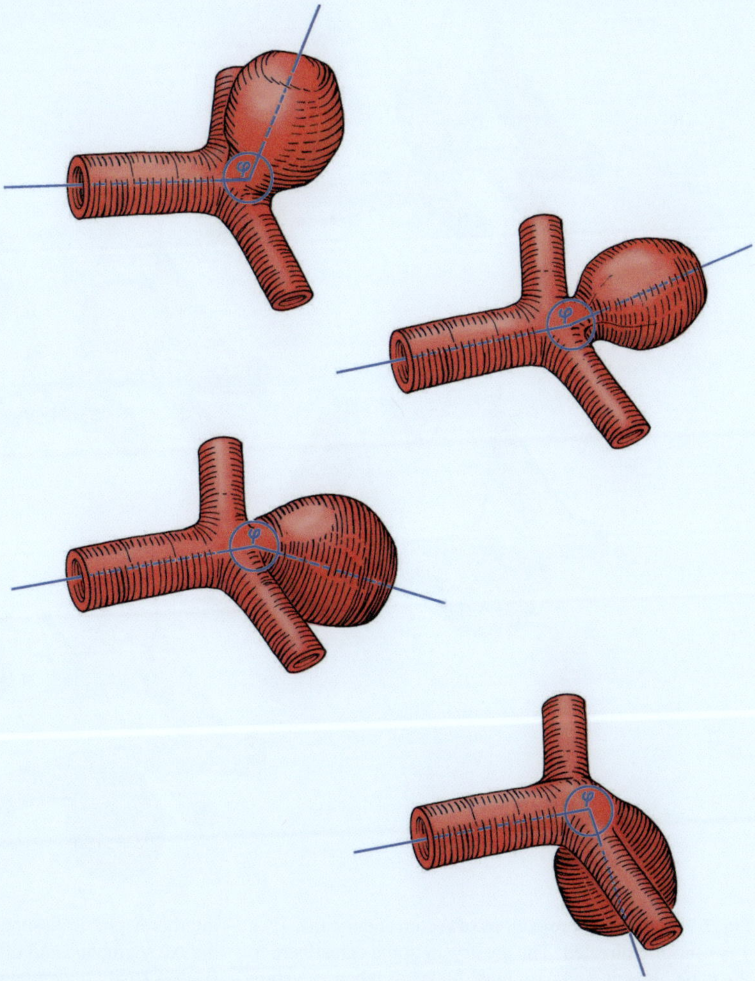

Fig. 2.8 Dominant aneurysm projections: A few typical aneurysm projections probably reflect a stable flow pattern. For MCA and Acom aneurysms, the typical angles between the axis of the afferent artery and the axis of the aneurysm are about 110° or about 160–170°

Based on measurements of the angles between the afferent artery and aneurysm projection on angiograms, we found that for the anterior communicating and middle cerebral aneurysm, two angles appear to be typical: one at about 110° and one at about 160–170° (Fig. 2.8). In reality, the measured angles scatter around these principal values because asymmetry of the outflow and the curvature of the aneurysmal plane also influence the flow pattern.

Since the dominant angles may be upward or downward, a total of four dominant aneurysm projections are observed, resulting in four typical configurations of the aneurysm location. These basic types are relevant for the microsurgical technique of aneurysm elimination, as they determine the approach, proximal vascular control, and the optimal application of the aneurysm clip or clips.

In the case of the anterior communicating artery aneurysm (Fig. 2.9), type 1 is ventrally directed. The aneurysm dome can adhere to the optic chiasm. When these type 1 aneurysms are approached, care is required to avoid tearing the dome off the chiasm when elevating the frontal lobe. Type 2 Acom aneurysms are directed anteriorly within the interhemispheric fissure. Here, the danger consists of tearing the dome when splitting the ventral interhemispheric fissure. Type 3 Acom aneurysms lie behind the plane of the A2 segments. The notion that the larger part of the aneurysm neck is on the back side is important when applying the aneurysm clip. Wrongly assuming that the neck looks the same on the back

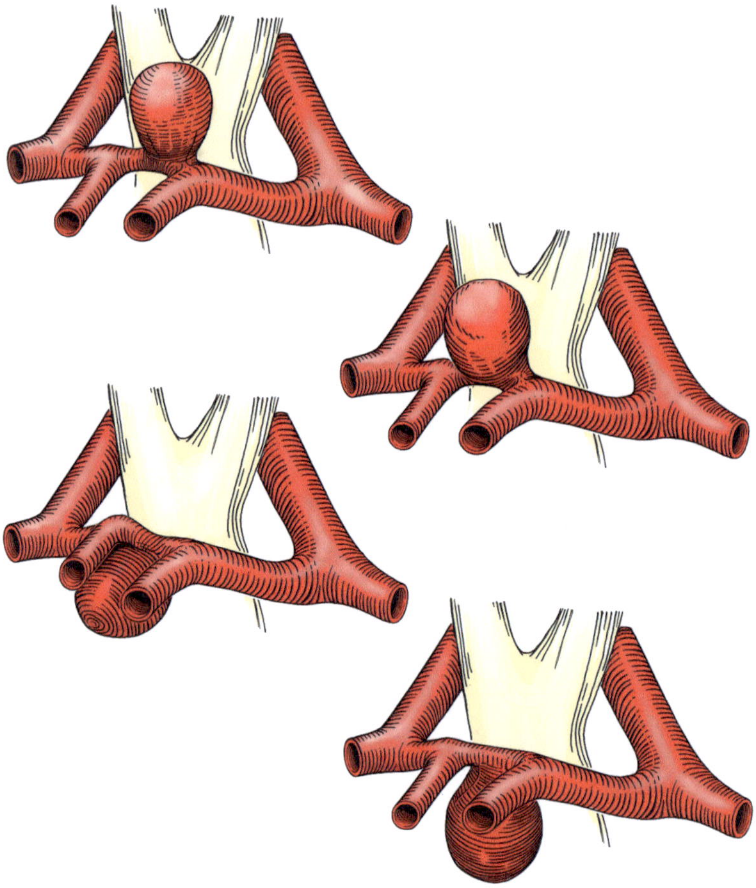

Fig. 2.9 Dominant projections of Acom aneurysms: *Type 1* is ventrally directed. The aneurysm dome can adhere to the optic chiasm, and care must be taken when elevating the orbital cortex during approach. *Type 2* is directed anteriorly within the interhemispheric fissure. Here, the danger consists of tearing the dome when splitting the ventral interhemispheric fissure. *Type 3* lies behind the plane of the A2 segments, and often the posterior part of the aneurysm is easily underestimated when it is approached from the front. *Type 4* projects upward, and these aneurysms require dissection above the A1 and behind the A2 segments

side as the visible anterior aspect would result in incomplete clipping of the posterior aspect. Finally, type 4 ACA aneurysms project upward. These aneurysms require dissection above the A1 segment and behind the A2 segment.

There are also different types of MCA bifurcation aneurysms (Fig. 2.10). Type 1 aneurysms are directed ventrally toward the temporal pole. These aneurysms often present with a temporal intracerebral hematoma. This notion is important in case of temporal mass hemorrhage presenting with coma and possibly mydriasis. The urgency for surgical evacuation does not allow detailed diagnostics such as angiography, but knowing that an aneurysm with a temporal projection (type 1) must be expected, with a diameter usually greater than 8 mm, suffices for safely approaching the aneurysm without angiography.

Type 2 MCA aneurysms lie in the Sylvian fissure in front of the plane of the M2 segments. Type 3 aneurysms are directed slightly medially. They lie between the M2 trunks and can be adherent to the insula. Type 4 MCA aneurysms are directed upward toward the frontal lobe.

For both ACA and MCA aneurysms, types 1 and 2 account for about 80 % of all aneurysms in these locations. This fact is probably related to the curved plane of the bifurcations, where aneurysms develop preferentially on the outer surface of the bifurcation plane.

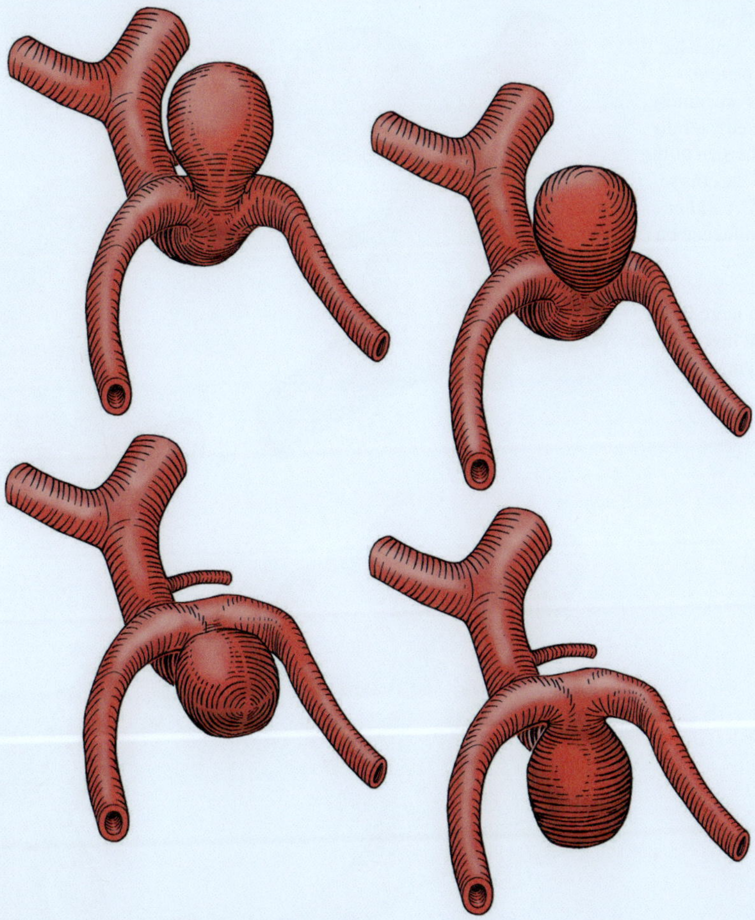

Fig. 2.10 Dominant projections of MCA aneurysms. *Type 1* MCA aneurysms are directed ventrally toward the temporal pole and can present with a temporal lobe hematoma. *Type 2* MCA aneurysms lie in the Sylvian fissure in front of the plane of the M2 segments. *Type 3* aneurysms are directed slightly medially. They lie between the M2 trunks and can be adherent to the insula. *Type 4* MCA aneurysms project upward toward the frontal lobe. They are rare

ICA posterior communicating artery (Pcom) aneurysms differ somewhat from the typical pattern. The anatomical restraints of the tentorial edge confine aneurysm growth to some degree. These aneurysms are almost universally directed laterally or posteriorly (Fig. 2.11); medial projections are hardly ever seen. There are medially oriented aneurysms of the distal ICA, but these back-wall aneurysms are not seen in the context of the Pcom origin. Because of the anatomical restraints, the typical angles between the afferent artery and the aneurysm projection are not seen with the ICA–Pcom aneurysm; instead, the angles are scattered around an average of about 110° [10].

On the other hand, the size of the Pcom influences the course of the terminal ICA and therefore has some influence on the projection of the aneurysm. ICA aneurysms associated with a large Pcom tend to have a more lateral projection. Therefore, we subdivide the Pcom aneurysms into types 1A and 2A, associated with a small Pcom, and types 1B and 2B, associated with a large Pcom or fetal origin of the posterior cerebral artery (2 mm or larger). In general, type 1 projection corresponds to a posterior and slightly lateral aneurysm of the ICA, whereas type 2 aneurysms project clearly laterally beneath the tentorial edge or, in rare cases, above the tentorial edge.

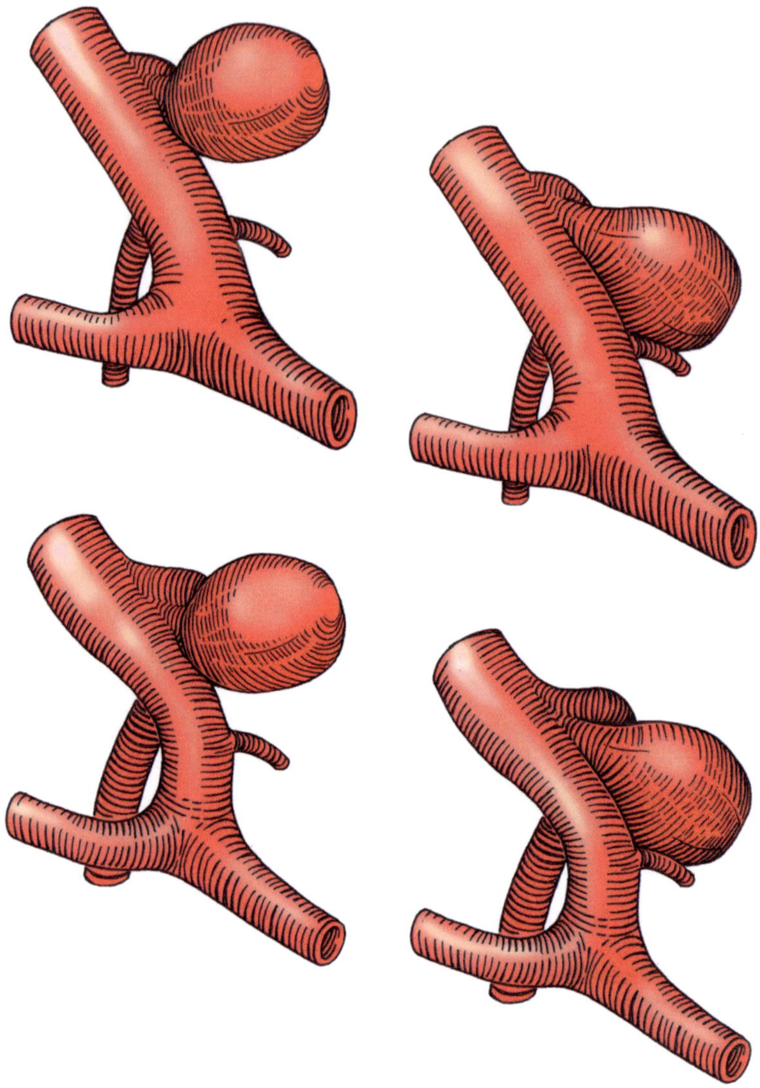

Fig. 2.11 ICA–Pcom aneurysms differ somewhat from the typical pattern. These aneurysms are almost universally directed laterally or posteriorly. The size of the Pcom influences the course of the terminal ICA and has therefore some influence on the projection of the aneurysm. Aneurysms associated with a large Pcom project somewhat higher than aneurysms involving a small Pcom branch

This latter constellation is seen more often with type 2B than 1B, because of the somewhat higher orientation of the bifurcation.

The projection above the tentorial edge brings the aneurysm dome into direct relation with the parahippocampal gyrus. In rare cases, these aneurysms become symptomatic with epilepsy. This constellation is not seen exclusively with posterior communicating artery aneurysms, but also occurs with aneurysms at the origin of the anterior choroidal artery.

In principle, the concept of dominant projections also applies to the other typical aneurysm sites: ICA and basilar bifurcation, A2-callosomarginal artery bifurcation, and posterior inferior cerebellar artery (PICA) origin. In case of the basilar bifurcation, all four typical projections are seen, with the anterior projections being more frequent. The case of the terminal ICA bifurcation is special, in that the projections are almost exclusively upward. With the more peripheral aneurysms and the aneurysms with PICA origin, on the other hand, the variability of the parent artery is relatively high, which transfers to a large variability of the orientation of the aneurysms. In the case of PICA aneurysms, the origin of this artery from the vertebral artery varies over a distance of several centimeters.

2.4 Shape of Aneurysm Necks

Aneurysms most often originate as punctate herniations of the intima through the tunica media. This primitive form is still apparent in the so-called blister-like aneurysms, which consist essentially of only an intimal layer and an adventitial layer. Later in the development, fibroblasts produce collagen that leads to temporary stability. Collagen alone is a viscoelastic substance that yields slowly to constant tension [11]. Therefore, long-term vascular stability is established only by the smooth muscle in the tunica media, but because aneurysm walls remain devoid of smooth muscle, slow growth must be assumed to take place in all aneurysms.

Interestingly, it is not rare for blister-like aneurysms leading to subarachnoid hemorrhage to be seen away from the typical aneurysm sites, particularly on the upper and medial wall of the ICA. It can be hypothesized that unusual mechanisms are involved in the genesis of these blister-like aneurysms, such as acute focal necrosis or inflammation in the tunica media.

Another somewhat enigmatic question is whether the funnel-like dilatations of the origin of branches (infundibula) play a role in the initial aneurysmal evolution. These infundibula occur particularly at the origin of the posterior communicating artery. The role of the infundibula in the development of the ICA–Pcom aneurysm remains hypothetical; it is suggested by a number of case reports in the literature, but nothing more.

In the initial stages of aneurysm development, neither the surrounding arterial wall nor the shape of the bifurcation is affected (Fig. 2.12). With further growth, the origin of the side branch becomes affected and eventually is integrated into the aneurysm neck. In the case of a lateral aneurysm, the next stage leads to involvement of the entire contour of the parent artery.

The sequence of events in the development of typical bifurcation aneurysms is comparable (Fig. 2.13). The only difference is that involvement of the two branches occurs more simultaneously. At the final stage, both branches appear to originate from the aneurysm neck, and the afferent artery becomes dilated.

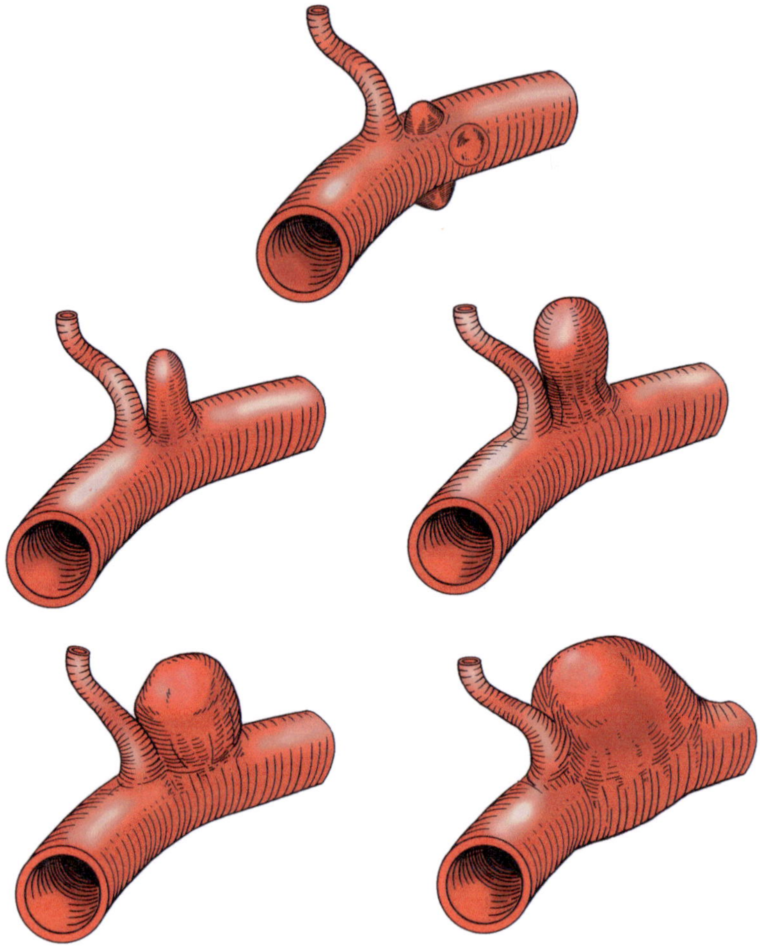

Fig. 2.12 Shape of aneurysm necks at different stages of side branch-related aneurysms: In the initial stages of aneurysm development, neither the surrounding arterial wall nor the shape of the bifurcation is affected. With further growth, the origin of the side branch becomes affected and eventually is integrated into the aneurysm neck. In the case of a lateral aneurysm, the next stage involves the entire contour of the parent artery

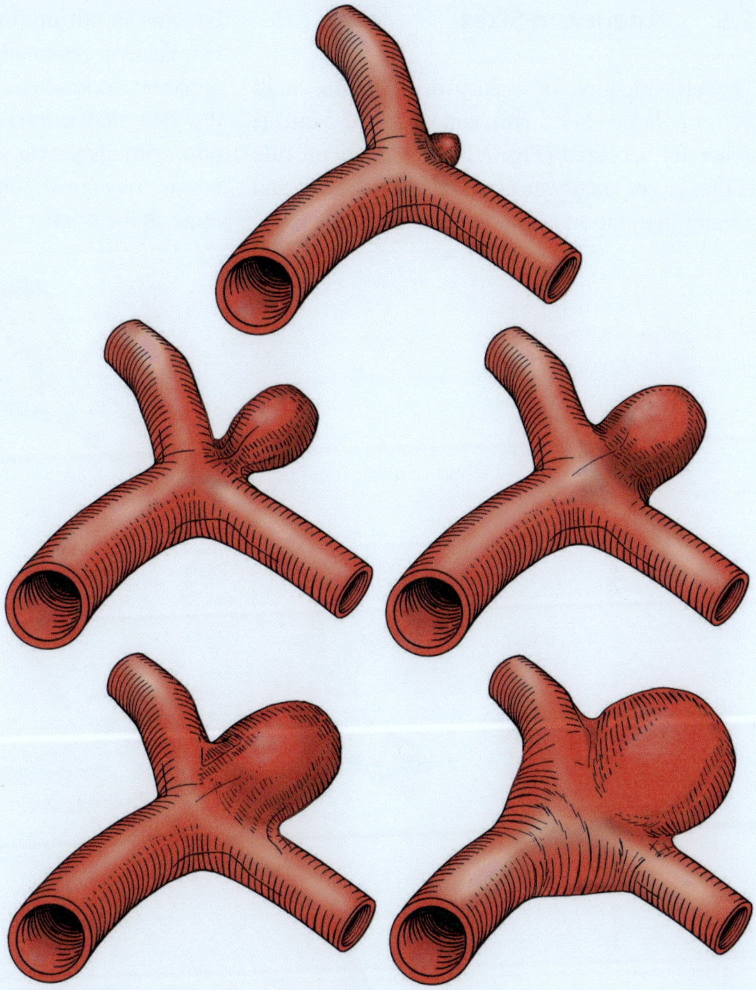

Fig. 2.13 Different stages of terminal aneurysms. In the beginning, neither the surrounding arterial wall nor the shape of the bifurcation is affected. At the final stage, both branches appear to originate from the aneurysm neck and the afferent artery becomes dilated

2.5 Aneurysm Sizes

The classification of aneurysm size into small (<1 cm), large (1–2.5 cm), and giant (>2.5 cm) is generally accepted (Fig. 2.14). The general rule is that larger aneurysms have a broader neck and greater integration of the branches into the neck, but this is not uniformly the case. Giant aneurysms are occasionally seen with a small neck, an apparent contradiction that can be explained by the fact that aneurysm growth may not occur homogenously over the entire wall. Some aneurysms may grow more at the neck, and others more at the dome.

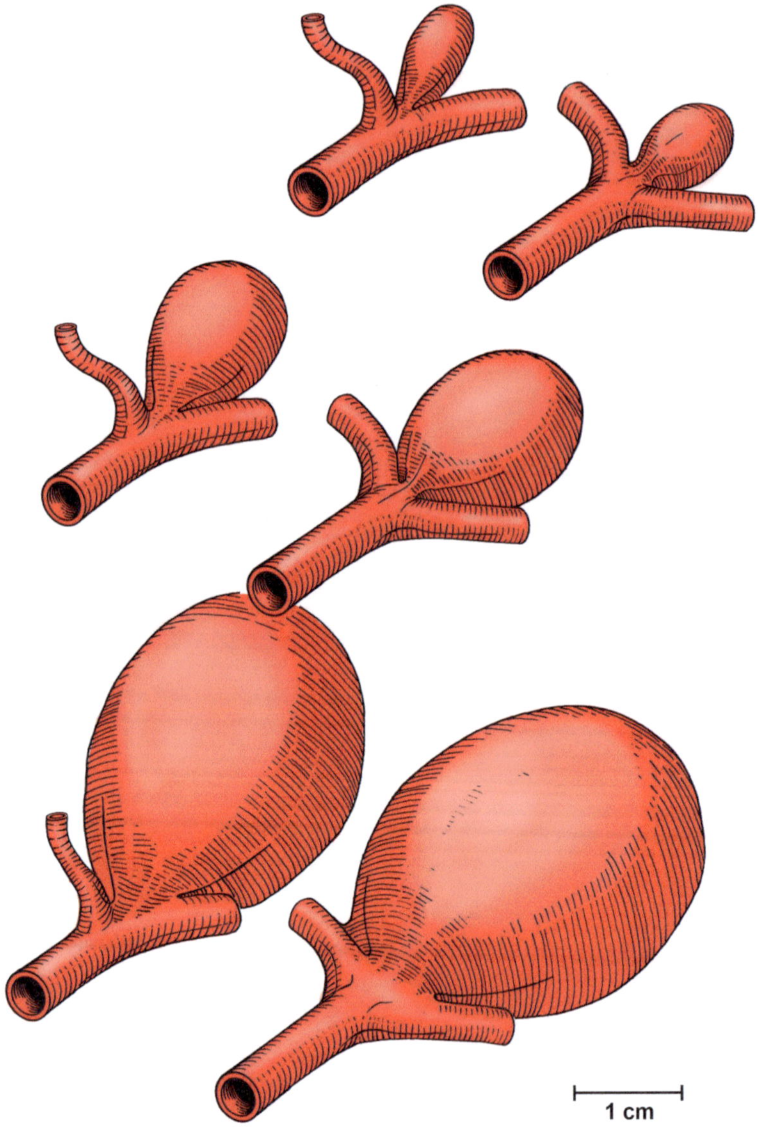

Fig. 2.14 Aneurysm sizes. The classification of aneurysm sizes into small (<1 cm), large (1–2.5 cm), and giant (>2.5 cm) is generally accepted. Although larger aneurysms generally have broader necks, a large aneurysm can have a small neck if growth takes place predominantly near the dome

2.6 Aneurysm Contours

Aneurysms differ in shape. Some are round, some pear shaped. Some have a relatively small neck and others a broad one. Some aneurysms have a smooth surface, but others develop small daughter aneurysms (Fig. 2.15). Some aspects of shape have been described as risk factors for rupture, such as the existence of daughter aneurysms or the aspect ratio, which defines the relation between height and neck width [12].

Ujiie et al. [12] found that the aspect ratio differed significantly between ruptured aneurysms and unruptured aneurysms: Almost 80 % of the ruptured aneurysms showed an aspect ratio of more than 1.6, whereas almost 90 % of the unruptured aneurysms had an aspect ratio of less than 1.6. These authors concluded that the aspect ratio of incidental aneurysms should be considered a risk factor for subsequent rupture and therefore potentially integrated into decision making, but this conclusion must be questioned. An alternative explanation for the different aspect ratios of ruptured and unruptured aneurysms is that the aspect ratio increases in context with the process of rupture, during which the aneurysms expand at the top. The difficulty addressed here applies also to other potential risk factors predicting the risk of rupture of unruptured aneurysms by comparison of the two cohorts. The large prospective trials on unruptured intracranial aneurysms mainly have defined size as a certain and significant risk factor [13, 14]. The Unruptured Cerebral Aneurysm Study of Japan (UCAS Japan) [14] was able to provide some evidence for the Japanese population that aneurysms with a daughter sac are also more likely to rupture (hazard ratio, 1.63; 95 % CI, 1.08–2.48).

Differences in the risk of rupture related to specific locations are also worth mentioning. The recent UCAS Japan trial [14] convincingly showed that anterior and posterior communicating artery aneurysms and basilar top aneurysms carry a clearly higher risk than MCA aneurysms, even as vertebral artery aneurysms have a lower risk.

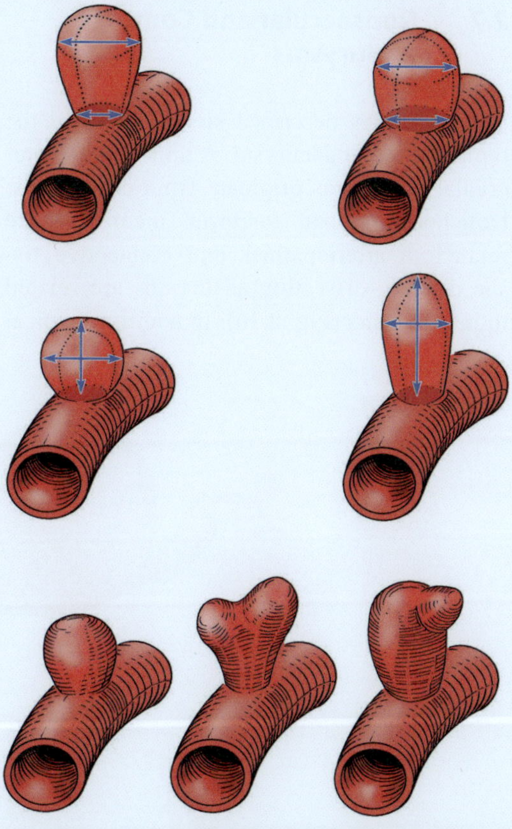

Fig. 2.15 Aneurysm contours. The neck-to-dome ratio separates aneurysms with a wide neck from those with a narrow neck. The relative width of the neck is important for endovascular coiling and also to some degree for microsurgical clipping. The aspect ratio defines the relation between the height and the width of the aneurysm. An aspect ratio of more than 1.6 is commonly found with ruptured aneurysms but rarely with unruptured aneurysms. Surface irregularities and daughter aneurysms also develop progressively during aneurysm evolution. When found with unruptured aneurysms, they are considered a risk factor for subsequent rupture

The neck-to-dome ratio is another relation defining aneurysm shape. It is defined as the relation of the diameters of the neck and the dome. In other words, the neck-to-dome ratio separates aneurysms with a wide neck from those with a narrow neck. The relative width of the neck is obviously important for endovascular coiling, but it is also somewhat important for microsurgical clipping.

2.7 Nonsaccular and Complex Aneurysms

The principles described so far relate to the typical saccular aneurysm. A minority of intracranial aneurysms originate from other roots: Dolichoectatic and fusiform aneurysms are related to arteriopathies and connective tissue disease; dissecting aneurysms are related to intimal tears (Fig. 2.16). In addition, typical saccular aneurysms can develop toward broad-based and almost fusiform shapes. From a more practical point of view, all these atypical configurations are summarized as complex aneurysms. Complex intracranial aneurysms include those classified as giant and those located in brain regions that are technically difficult to access or those that involve arterial trunks and branches and/or have complicated wall structure.

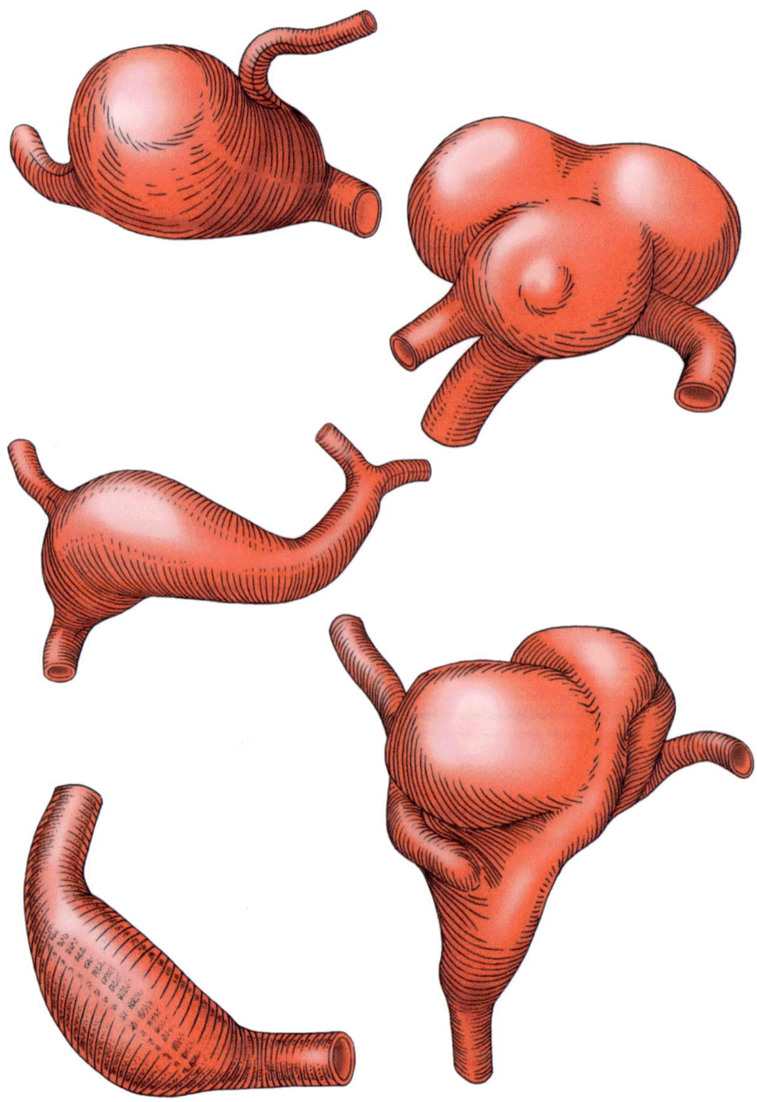

Fig. 2.16 Different faces of complex aneurysms: giant and broad-based, dolichoectatic and fusiform, and dissecting

References

1. Sahs AL, Perret GF, Locksley HB, Nishioka H. Intracranial aneurysm and subarachnoid hemorrhage. Report of the Cooperative Study. Philadelphia: JB Lippincott; 1969.
2. Yasargil MG. Microneurosurgery, vol. 1. Stuttgart: Thieme; 1984.
3. Suzuki M, Fujisawa H, Ishihara H, Yoneda H, Kato S, Ogawa A. Side selection of pterional approach for anterior communicating artery aneurysms–surgical anatomy and strategy. Acta Neurochir (Wien). 2008;150:31–9; discussion 39.
4. Huber P, Braun J, Hirschmann D, Agyeman JF. Incidence of berry aneurysms of the unpaired pericallosal artery: angiographic study. Neuroradiology. 1980;19:143–7.
5. Kirgis HD, Fisher WL, Llewellyn RC, Peebles EM. Aneurysms of the anterior communicating artery and gross anomalies of the circle of Willis. J Neurosurg. 1966;25:73–8.
6. Kayembe KN, Sasahara M, Hazama F. Cerebral aneurysms and variations in the circle of Willis. Stroke. 1984;15:846–50.
7. Matsuda M, Handa J, Saito A, Matsuda I, Kamijyo Y. Ruptured cerebral aneurysms associated with arterial occlusion. Surg Neurol. 1983;20:4–12.
8. Hodgson TJ, Zaman SM, Cooper JR, Forster DM. Proximal aneurysms in association with arteriovenous malformations: do they resolve following obliteration of the malformation with stereotactic radiosurgery? Br J Neurosurg. 1998;12:434–7.
9. Meisel HJ, Mansmann U, Alvarez H, Rodesch G, Brock M, Lasjaunias P. Cerebral arteriovenous malformations and associated aneurysms: analysis of 305 cases from a series of 662 patients. Neurosurgery. 2000;46:793–800; discussion 800–2.
10. Steiger HJ. Pathophysiology of development and rupture of cerebral aneurysms. Acta Neurochir Suppl (Wien). 1990;48:1–57.
11. Steiger HJ, Aaslid R, Keller S, Reulen HJ. Strength, elasticity and viscoelastic properties of cerebral aneurysms. Heart Vessels. 1989;5:41–6.
12. Ujiie H, Tachibana H, Hiramatsu O, Hazel AL, Matsumoto T, Ogasawara Y, et al. Effects of size and shape (aspect ratio) on the hemodynamics of saccular aneurysms: a possible index for surgical treatment of intracranial aneurysms. Neurosurgery. 1999;45:119–29; discussion 129–30.
13. Wiebers DO, Whisnant JP, Huston 3rd J, Meissner I, Brown Jr RD, Piepgras DG, et al.; International Study of Unruptured Intracranial Aneurysms Investigators. Unruptured intracranial aneurysms: natural history, clinical outcome, and risks of surgical and endovascular treatment. Lancet. 2003;362:103–10.
14. UCAS Japan Investigators, Morita A, Kirino T, Hashi K, Aoki N, Fukuhara S, et al. The natural course of unruptured cerebral aneurysms in a Japanese cohort. N Engl J Med. 2012;366:2474–82.

3 Perioperative Management of Patients with Subarachnoid Hemorrhage

3.1 Guidelines for the Admission

Transport to the neurosurgical center and preoperative diagnostics of patients in good grade after subarachnoid hemorrhage (SAH) should always be organized in an efficient—but not rushed—manner. It is advisable to admit all patients with suspected or proven SAH without undue delay. We do not recommend initiation of treatment and angiography in peripheral hospitals that are not equipped for surgical management of aneurysms. This general policy admittedly depends to some degree on local circumstances. Patients with space-occupying intracranial hematoma present an emergency situation that requires immediate action. The same applies to all SAH patients with ventricular hemorrhage, early hydrocephalus, or both. All poor-grade patients should be transferred to the center, because early optimization of cerebral perfusion and intracranial pressure appears to be critical for recovery.

On the other hand, we do not recommend rushing good-grade patients to the center on an emergency basis. It is well known that about 10 % of patients suffer a rebleed on day 0. We also know that angiography during the first 6 h after SAH is complicated by a rebleed in up to 20 % of patients. Therefore stabilization of the patient with analgesia, slight sedation, and blood pressure control is of primary importance during the first hours after SAH. Transport and angiography should be planned for the second half of day zero.

3.2 Initial Assessment

3.2.1 Clinical Examination

We prefer to use the World Federation of Neurosurgical Societies (WFNS) scale (Table 3.1), which is based on the Glasgow Coma Scale (GCS), to evaluate the patient's initial clinical condition (i.e., state of consciousness and focal neurologic deficits) [1]. The WFNS score during day zero is not a static entity, but is influenced by multiple factors. In approximately half of all patients, SAH is accompanied by coma; in about half of this group, the coma is transient. Depending on the time of assessment, the momentary responsiveness does not adequately reflect the impact of SAH. Early hydrocephalus also leads secondarily to significant functional depression within the first hours or days. Therefore, the course of the WFNS score over the initial day must be evaluated for a prognostic estimate.

The overall clinical assessment must include additional general medical risk factors, which are

Table 3.1 The WFNS grading scale

	GCS	Focal deficit[a]
Grade I	15	No
Grade II	13–14	No
Grade III	13–14	Yes
Grade IV	7–12	Yes or no
Grade V	3–6	Yes or no

GCS Glasgow Coma Scale, *WFNS* World Federation of Neurosurgical Societies
[a]Aphasia and/or hemiparesis

H.-J. Steiger et al., *Microsurgical Brain Aneurysms: Illustrated Concepts and Cases*,
DOI 10.1007/978-3-662-45679-8_3, © Springer-Verlag Berlin Heidelberg 2015

well known to influence outcome. Prognostic factors that are especially unfavorable in aneurysm patients include hypertension, diabetes, coronary heart disease, use of an oral anticoagulant, or advanced age.

3.2.2 Computed Tomography

Initial ancillary tests should include standard blood laboratory tests and cranial computed tomography (CCT) for localization and assessment of the extent of hemorrhage (Fisher Grading Scale, Table 3.2) [2]. After 4–5 days, the blood in the basal cisterns becomes isodense, and SAH is no longer detectable by CCT in some 50 % of cases. In these patients, a spinal tap is necessary to detect xanthochromic cerebrospinal fluid (CSF). Traces of the SAH can be detected in the CSF up to 4 weeks after hemorrhage.

If neurologic deterioration occurs after the initial CT scan, the exam must be repeated to rule out a rerupture or hydrocephalus.

3.2.3 Cerebral Perfusion Monitoring

We recommend baseline assessment and monitoring of cerebral perfusion and vasospasm with transcranial Doppler sonography (TCD) and perfusion CT (pCT). Both methods are semiquantitative tools with limited sensitivity and specificity. To get the maximum from TCD, it is important to thoroughly examine the intracranial arteries and also investigate the high cervical internal carotid artery (ICA) to appreciate overall hemispheric perfusion and determine the Lindegaard index (blood velocity in the middle cerebral artery [vMCA] divided by the velocity in the ipsilateral ICA [vICA]) [3]. Lindegaard indices greater than 3 denote vasospasm. TCD should be performed daily during the first week and then depending on the clinical course. Perfusion CT should not be done daily, owing to the necessary exposure to radiation and contrast medium. We recommend routine performance of an initial baseline exam and then one or two follow-up studies during the first 10 days. Additional exams must be performed in patients with secondary neurologic deterioration.

Table 3.2 Modified Fisher SAH grading on CT

Grade	Blood visible on CT scan
Grade 0	None
Grade 1	Local thin blood film
Grade 2	Diffuse thin SAH (<1 mm)
Grade 3	Cisternal tamponade (>1 mm, local or diffuse)
Grade 4	Ventricular or intraparenchymal hemorrhage with or without SAH

The original scale from the late 1970s no longer reflects the current resolution of CT scanning
CT computed tomography, *SAH* subarachnoid hemorrhage

3.2.4 Angiography

Panangiography should be planned for clinically stable patients within 24 h after admission, but it should be avoided within the first 6 h after the initial ictus because of a high risk of rerupture [4]. We do not recommend angiography during the night in stable patients admitted late. In these cases, CT angiography can be considered to be an exploratory investigation.

3.2.5 Exceptions

Panangiography should be dispensed with in emergencies with intracerebral mass hemorrhage and impending transtentorial herniation. We recommend giving these patients mannitol (1–2 g/kg body weight) and taking them immediately to the operating room following CT, which always can be completed by a contrast angiography series. Space-occupying intracerebral mass bleeding most often results from MCA aneurysms or less frequently from anterior communicating artery aneurysms. Acute subdural hematoma usually results from ICA–posterior communicating artery (Pcom) aneurysms.

The management of patients with early ventricular dilatation on CT must remain individualized, depending on the state of consciousness. If the state of consciousness is marginal or deteriorating, external CSF drainage should be installed prior to angiography.

3.3 Choice of Treatment Modality and Timing of Securing the Aneurysm

Following angiography, interdisciplinary consultation between the neurosurgeon and the endovascular therapist must define the optimal mode of securing the aneurysm. The decision will usually include aneurysm factors and specifics of the hemorrhage (i.e., whether surgical evacuation of a hematoma or decompression may be desirable), as well as logistical aspects such as the available endovascular and neurosurgical competence. The interdisciplinary conference usually must result in a clear recommendation to the patient, but it would be an illusion to assume that the patient, usually still lying in the angiography suite, is in a position to make an informed decision at this time.

If endovascular therapy is planned, the patient usually undergoes treatment immediately following the decision. Patients in good clinical grades (WFNS I–III) stratified for microsurgical clipping should be taken to the operating room at the first logistically convenient time within 24 h after the hemorrhage or admission.

Patients in poor clinical grades (WFNS IV–V) without space-occupying hematoma should be equipped with ventriculostomy prior to angiography and, if possible, endovascular treatment. If intracranial pressure is stable, angiography and coiling (or, if that is not possible, clipping) should also be planned within 24 h. If initial recordings of intracranial pressure show persistently elevated values (≥30 mmHg), a fatal outcome cannot be avoided and going ahead with angiography and aneurysm elimination is not recommended [5].

3.4 Initial Management (Before Elimination of Aneurysm)

3.4.1 General Measures

Avoidance of rerupture is the primary objective following hospital admission. Patients with WFNS grades II or higher are optimally cared for in the ICU, but Grade I patients are more comfortable in a quiet room on the normal ward.

Stress avoidance is more important than recording vital signs and checking neurologic status. Stress reduction should include relative bed rest. Getting up to go to the toilet is associated with less stress than not getting up. Visits from relatives and friends should be restricted to the closest family members. Smoking, watching television, and using phones and computers are typically not recommended.

Analgesia for headache with paracetamol or other oral drugs, mild sedation, and stool softeners should be prescribed prophylactically. Injections should be avoided.

In unstable, comatose, or uncooperative patients, insertion of a central venous line is necessary before angiography. Otherwise, a central venous line can be inserted together with induction of anesthesia for surgery or endovascular therapy.

Patients who have been intubated for transport or medical procedures after admission should not be extubated until the ruptured aneurysm has been secured.

Total fluid intake orally or via infusion should amount to about 3,000 mL/day.

We recommend giving corticosteroids (e.g., dexamethasone 3×4 mg p.o./IV), although their effect remains a matter of discussion. A possibly protective effect with regard to vasospasm and cerebral edema remains unproven, but we believe that the obvious reduction of meningeal irritation and headache effect justifies prescribing them during the first week following SAH.

A gastric antacid such as ranitidine should be prescribed prophylactically. However, the interaction of omeprazole with clopidogrel and similar drugs should be kept in mind. Loss of the clopidogrel effect has been reported in patients using omeprazole.

Nimodipine has been proven effective to prevent and treat clinical sequels of cerebral vasospasm [6, 7]. Oral administration of 6×60 mg/day is recommended for good-grade patients. Intravenous (IV) administration is necessary for unconscious patients. The dose should be gradually increased over 12 h to 2 mg/h. The dose needs to be reduced for patients weighing less than

60 kg or if arterial hypotension ensues (<110 mg systolic).

3.4.2 Analgesia and Sedation

Potent analgesics and sedatives should be given only under monitored conditions, particularly when administered intravenously.

The doses given are intended as a guide. In the ICU, appropriate sedation and analgesia can be given according to the local standard (e.g., with fentanyl or sufentanil).

Treatment of headache should precede sedation. We recommend oral paracetamol up to 6×500 mg, with oral morphine (2–6×10–30 mg) as second-line therapy.

Some degree of sedation should be aimed at. Patients should be calm but awake and assessable. Diazepam (Valium®) is usually effective and well tolerated at an oral dose of up to 3×5–10 mg/day. Slow IV administration at a dose of up to 3×2–5 mg/day is also possible. The effect must be monitored carefully; the long half-life (20–40 h) makes it difficult to control. Side effects include respiratory depression, hypotension, and paradoxical reaction, especially in elderly patients.

For younger patients, clorazepate at an oral or IV dose of 3×5–10 mg is a good alternative for benzodiazepines. For older patients (particularly those who are hypertensive), clonidine can be a good alternative, given at a dosage up to 4×0.15 mg (oral or IV).

3.4.3 Blood Pressure Control

Before securing the aneurysm, arterial hypertension must be controlled pharmacologically, with systolic blood pressure limits of 140 mmHg in previously normotensive patients and 160 mmHg in known hypertensive patients. The first step should be to ensure adequate analgesia and sedation and to increase IV nimodipine to 3 mg/h. Further antihypertensive therapy can be done with oral nifedipine (3–4×20 mg) or oral or IV urapidil or clonidine.

Hypotension also must be avoided during the initial phase. For systolic arterial pressure less than 100 mmHg (or <120 mmHg in known hypertensive patients), intravenous infusion should be increased to a rate of 150 mL/h and IV nimodipine should be reduced to 1–1.5 mg/h.

Colloidal solutions such as hydroxyethyl starch (HES) can also be used to increase plasma volume, although the position of the colloidal infusions is debated [8]. Inotropic drugs such as epinephrine or norepinephrine must be considered dangerous in patients with unsecured aneurysms and should be given only in exceptional cases in the ICU.

3.5 Preoperative Measures

For aneurysm microsurgery, lumbar CSF drainage is placed after induction of anesthesia in patients with recent SAH without space-occupying hemorrhage, unless ventriculostomy has previously been placed. Following craniotomy and opening of the dura, 50–100 mL of CSF should be drained.

A sufficient level of anesthesia must have been obtained prior to fixation of the Mayfield clamp. We recommend mannitol at a dose of 1.0 g/kg for early surgery after SAH, except in elderly patients, in whom the dosage should be reduced or none should be given.

3.6 Postoperative Treatment

3.6.1 Medication and Fluid Therapy

Sufficient hydration (at least 3 L/day) is important in order to optimize cerebral perfusion. Oral intake must be supplemented with electrolyte or colloidal infusion, although there are currently some uncertainties with regard to the pros and cons of colloidal infusion.

We recommend, in addition, standard thromboprophylaxis with low-molecular-weight heparin at a dosage of 20 mg/day or 40 mg in patients weighing over 70 kg or at risk (bedridden or with hemiparesis).

Dexamethasone should be weaned from the initial dose of 3×4 mg/day within the first week. Nimodipine should be continued for at least 1 week and then gradually reduced in the absence of clinical or instrumentally detected vasospasm. In patients with signs of vasospasm, nimodipine should be maintained throughout the phase of vasospasm but maximally for 3 weeks. If sonographic vasospasm or prolongation of mean transit time (MTT) above 4 s is seen in perfusion CT, IV nimodipine should be continued until the MCA flow velocities drop below 120 cm/s and MTT is below 4 s. If the TCD values stay above 120 cm/s 3 weeks after SAH, the medication can be weaned without danger. The current understanding is that such fixed spasm is no longer critical and will resolve after a period of 1–2 months.

Nimodipine was proven effective in the management of subarachnoid hemorrhage at an oral dose of 6×60 mg/day [9, 10]. The data regarding IV nimodipine were less convincing, partially because of the quality of the studies. It is also possible that the negative effect on blood pressure partially canceled the positive effects. Nonetheless, IV use has many advantages over oral administration, particularly in the immediate perioperative period and in poor-grade patients. We prefer intravenous application during the early management of SAH, but it is important to control arterial pressure carefully. The standard dose of 2 mg/h should be achieved gradually, starting with an initial dose of 1.0 mg/h for 6 h. If hypotension (systolic blood pressure <110 mmHg) should ensue at the standard dose, reduction to 1 or 1.5 mg/h should be done. Dose reduction is also necessary in patients weighing less than 60 kg.

Nimodipine occasionally leads to damage of the pancreas, liver, or both, so enzymes must be controlled at least weekly.

Although we do not recommend prophylactic hypertensive management following clipping or coiling, maintaining high normal blood pressures is important to minimize the risk of ischemic deficits. We recommend keeping systolic blood pressures above 120 mmHg in normotensive patients (mean arterial pressure [MAP] >80 mmHg) and above 130 mmHg in hypertensive patients (MAP >90 mmHg). In hypertensive patients, the antihypertensive medication brought from home is discontinued during the early postoperative phase.

In case of symptomatic vasospasm, induced hypertension is the basis of treatment. Positive inotropic drugs must be used at this stage, aiming at systolic blood pressures of up to 200 mmHg.

3.6.2 Controls

We recommend the following schedule for ancillary examinations during the postoperative phase:

- TCD/cervical Doppler daily during the first week and additionally in case of delayed neurologic deficit.
- Hematology, renal, pancreatic, and hepatic and coagulation parameters on days 1, 3, and 7.
- Plain CT postoperatively and additionally in case of secondary focal neurologic deficit or decreasing level of consciousness.
- Perfusion CT on days 1, 3–4, and 9–11 and in case of delayed neurologic deficit.
- Control angiography between the 5th and 7th postoperative days. Routine control angiography at this time is not necessary if it was already done intraoperatively or immediately postoperatively.

3.6.3 Mobilization

Patients in good neurologic condition are mobilized postoperatively as soon as possible but only in the absence of evidence of vasospasm.

3.7 Treatment of Symptomatic Vasospasm

3.7.1 General Considerations

Symptomatic (clinical) and angiographic or sonographic vasospasm must be distinguished.

Symptomatic spasm must be treated immediately to prevent brain infarction. Symptoms such as clouding of consciousness, agitation, hemiparesis or monoparesis, and aphasic disorders are signs of vasospasms unless proven differently. The beginning of clinical vasospasm is often insidious, with headache, confusion, restlessness, or lethargy.

In contrast to the urgency associated with symptomatic vasospasm, asymptomatic spasm as detected by angiography, TCD, or perfusion CT calls only for precautionary measures (i.e., monitoring and optimization of blood pressure).

3.7.2 Diagnostics

TCD flow values greater than 140 cm/s or an increase greater than 30 cm/s within 24 h must be considered relevant. Indirect evidence for a segmental or peripheral vasospasm is a drop in the high cervical ICA flow velocity (normal, 35–45 cm/s) and an increase of the Lindegaard index to greater than 3.

CT perfusion has been more and more accepted as an additional tool to monitor vasospasm. The parameters are still less well standardized than the TCD parameters, and they apparently depend on the equipment and the exact setup. Mean transit time (MTT) appears to be the most sensitive surrogate parameter for cerebral perfusion in the setting of vasospasm. MTT values greater than 4 s are considered critical.

Plain CT remains important in the diagnosis of vasospasm in order to exclude other causes of secondary deterioration, such as hydrocephalus, swelling, infarction, rebleeding, and surgical complications.

Finally, blood laboratory and blood gas analysis are required to rule out electrolyte imbalance, especially hyponatremia but also hypoxia or hypercarbia.

3.7.3 Treatment of Symptomatic Vasospasm in the ICU

"Triple-H therapy" (hypervolemia, hemodilution, and hypertension) has been widely accepted as the most effective way of treating symptomatic vasospasm [11]. Blood pressure is the relevant parameter, and expansion of blood volume must be considered only a means to induce hypertension [12]. According to the severity of vasospasm (but also considering patient age and cardiopulmonary condition), systolic blood pressures between 150 and 220 mmHg are aimed at. As a rule of thumb, the maximum TCD flow velocity in centimeters per second is a good initial target value for the systolic blood pressure. The value of hemodilution per se has also been questioned. It is generally accepted that hemoglobin levels of about 10 g/100 mL (hematocrit 30–35 %) are a reasonable compromise with respect to blood viscosity and oxygen transport capacity. Hypervolemia should aim at a target central venous pressure of 6–10 mmHg. Plasma expansion is achieved by colloidal infusion, mainly with HES. Recent publications have demonstrated a negative impact of HES in other conditions, so it will need reevaluation in the management of vasospasm [8]. One aspect that is often ignored is the effect of hemodilution on TCD and perfusion CT. Under physiological conditions, perfusion is adjusted according to the oxygen transport capacity. Within the normal bandwidth of hematocrit levels, minor fluctuations need not be considered when judging TCD and perfusion CT. In contrast, major fluctuations such as a drop of the hemoglobin from 14 to 10 g per 100 mL must be compensated in consideration. With such a drop, TCD velocities would increase approximately 30 %, as would CBF parameters in perfusion CT, corresponding to a 30 % decrease of MTT.

Catecholamines usually must be added to bring hypertension to the desired level. Triple-H therapy therefore requires appropriate monitoring of blood pressure and systemic cardiovascular parameters, so transfer to the ICU or an appropriate intermediate-care ward is necessary

Adjuvant measures include strict bed rest. We recommend a slight head-up position of 10–30°.

Blood oxygenation must be watched. If the level of consciousness decreases, early intubation and ventilation (normoventilation) is recommended.

The installation of external CSF drainage to optimize cerebral perfusion should be considered early, particularly if increased intracranial pressure is suspected. Intracranial pressure should be reduced to 10–15 mmHg by draining CSF and by sedation. Nimodipine can be increased to an IV dosage of 2.5–3 mg/h if that does not interfere with the targeted blood pressures.

The value of corticosteroids in the situation of vasospasm is still debated. At the moment, there is not enough evidence to support their administration for the indication of vasospasm. As mentioned above, we add dexamethasone to the initial management of SAH to reduce meningeal irritation. Hydrocortisone or mineralosteroids have been used to increase plasma volume, but the benefit has not yet been conclusively proven [13].

Balloon angioplasty and intra-arterial nimodipine therapy should be considered if the above measures are insufficient—i.e., if delayed neurologic deficits persist or worsen under triple-H therapy or if perfusion CT indicates focal misery perfusion with MTT greater than 4 s. We recommend balloon angioplasty as the first choice of intra-arterial therapy for proximal and segmental spasms and nimodipine infusion for diffuse and more distal spasm.

It goes without saying that triple-H therapy cannot be used in patients with an unsecured ruptured aneurysm. Because most ruptured aneurysms are now referred early, however, symptomatic vasospasm is rarely seen in such patients.

A more burning question is what to do for a patient with multiple aneurysms after initial clipping or coiling of only some of the aneurysms (including the ruptured aneurysm, it is hoped). In this situation, we recommend not limiting triple-H therapy because of untreated incidental aneurysms. In other words, we recommend applying the same blood pressure targets in a patient with symptomatic vasospasm and one or more residual incidental aneurysms as for the patient with a single aneurysm that has been clipped or coiled. This policy leads to occasional disaster, but being reluctant with induced hypertension will lead to frequent disaster.

3.7.4 Management of Hydrocephalus

Approximately 25 % of all patients admitted with SAH finally need a ventriculoperitoneal shunt. The risk that poor-grade patients (with an initial WFNS grade of 12 or less) will become shunt-dependent is much higher than for initially good-grade patients. Among the good-grade patients, pronounced SAH appears to be the main determining factor for later shunt dependence. Advanced age is probably also associated with a higher risk of needing a shunt [14]. Efforts to remove intraventricular or subarachnoid blood by fibrinolysis or surgical cleansing have not been proven convincingly to reduce the risk of shunt dependence.

According to our outline policy, external ventriculostomy is done in all poor-grade patients upon admission. Following the acute phase, the amount of drainage is weaned, usually during the second week after the maximum of vasospastic cerebral ischemia has been passed. If weaning is unsuccessful, an internalized shunt should be placed without further delay. Even if weaning is initially successful and the external ventricular drain can be removed, the size of the ventricular system needs to be followed closely by means of CT. If the ventricles are enlarging, insertion of a shunt should not be postponed, even if the state of consciousness appears good.

We recommend the same policy for initially good-grade patients when CT indicates progressive hydrocephalus. Experience teaches that ventricular enlargement after SAH is not a spontaneously reversible condition, and delaying the indication for a ventriculoperitoneal shunt prolongs the overall time of recovery.

In patients with SAH-associated hydrocephalus, we recommend the use of valves with fixed settings. Patients readmitted for hydrocephalus weeks or months after the SAH are an exception. These patients exhibit the characteristics of normal pressure hydrocephalus instead, and the use of a programmable valve allows specific needs to be met properly.

3.8 Treatment of Patients with SAH Without an Angiographically Proven Source of Bleeding

The course following SAH is usually benign in patients with negative angiography. In general, the development of vasospasm and hydrocephalus is rare. We recommend progressive mobilization during the first week. Besides symptomatic medication for headache, we prescribe oral nimodipine at a dose of 6×60 mg for 1 week, with subsequent weaning. Sequential TCD exams are recommended during the first week because vasospasm, although rare, occurs occasionally.

Control angiography is required only for exceptional cases, such as qualitative defects of the first investigation, very massive SAH, or suspicious arterial segments. Blister-like aneurysms and dissecting aneurysms can be particularly difficult to identify on angiography, but these aneurysm types often change their shape rapidly, so that follow-up angiography can possibly visualize them better than did the initial study.

References

1. Teasdale GM, Drake CG, Hunt W, Kassell N, Sano K, Pertuiset B, et al. A universal subarachnoid hemorrhage scale: report of a committee of the World Federation of Neurosurgical Societies. J Neurol Neurosurg Psychiatry. 1988;51:1457.
2. Kistler JP, Crowell RM, Davis KR, Heros R, Ojemann RG, Zervas T, et al. The relation of cerebral vasospasm to the extent and location of subarachnoid blood visualized by CT scan: a prospective study. Neurology. 1983;33:424–36.
3. Lindegaard KF, Nornes H, Bakke SJ, Sorteberg W, Nakstad P. Cerebral vasospasm diagnosis by means of angiography and blood velocity measurements. Acta Neurochir (Wien). 1989;100:12–24.
4. Kusumi M, Yamada M, Kitahara T, Endo M, Kan S, Iida H, et al. Rerupture of cerebral aneurysms during angiography–a retrospective study of 13 patients with subarachnoid hemorrhage. Acta Neurochir (Wien). 2005;147:831–7.
5. Bailes JE, Spetzler RF, Hadley MN, Baldwin HZ. Management morbidity and mortality of poor-grade aneurysm patients. J Neurosurg. 1990;72:559–66.
6. Connolly Jr ES, Rabinstein AA, Carhuapoma JR, Derdeyn CP, Dion J, Higashida RT, et al. Guidelines for the management of aneurysmal subarachnoid hemorrhage: a guideline for healthcare professionals from the American Heart Association/American Stroke Association. Stroke. 2012;43:1711–37.
7. Diringer MN, Bleck TP, Claude Hemphill 3rd J, Menon D, Shutter L, Vespa P, et al. Critical care management of patients following aneurysmal subarachnoid hemorrhage: recommendations from the Neurocritical Care Society's Multidisciplinary Consensus Conference. Neurocrit Care. 2011;15:211–40.
8. Khan SA, Adogwa O, Gan TJ, Null UT, Verla T, Gokhale S, et al. Effect of 6 % hydroxyethyl starch 130/0.4 in 0.9 % sodium chloride (Voluven®) on complications after subarachnoid hemorrhage: a retrospective analysis. Springerplus. 2013;2:314.
9. Dorhout Mees SM, Rinkel GJ, Feigin VL, Algra A, van den Bergh WM, Vermeulen M, et al. Calcium antagonists for aneurysmal subarachnoid haemorrhage. Cochrane Database Syst Rev. 2007;(3):CD000277.
10. Feigin VL, Anderson N, Rinkel GJ, Algra A, van Gijn J, Bennett DA. Corticosteroids for aneurysmal subarachnoid haemorrhage and primary intracerebral haemorrhage. Cochrane Database Syst Rev. 2005;(3):CD004583.
11. Meyer R, Deem S, Yanez ND, Souter M, Lam A, Treggiari MM. Current practices of triple-H prophylaxis and therapy in patients with subarachnoid hemorrhage. Neurocrit Care. 2011;14:24–36.
12. Raabe A, Beck J, Keller M, Vatter H, Zimmermann M, Seifert V. Relative importance of hypertension compared with hypervolemia for increasing cerebral oxygenation in patients with cerebral vasospasm after subarachnoid hemorrhage. J Neurosurg. 2005;103:974–81.
13. Gomis P, Graftieaux JP, Sercombe R, Hettler D, Scherpereel B, Rousseaux P. Randomized, double-blind, placebo-controlled, pilot trial of high-dose methylprednisolone in aneurysmal subarachnoid hemorrhage. J Neurosurg. 2010;112:681–8.
14. Woernle CM, Winkler KM, Burkhardt JK, Haile SR, Bellut D, Neidert MC, et al. Hydrocephalus in 389 patients with aneurysm-associated subarachnoid hemorrhage. J Clin Neurosci. 2013;20:824–6.

4 Surgical Approaches

4.1 General Philosophy and Procedures

4.1.1 Approaches

In recent decades, the philosophy regarding approaches and adjuvant measures (i.e., imaging and planning tools and neurophysiological monitoring) has seen considerable changes. Following its formal description in the 1960s and 1970s, the pterional approach became standard for most anterior circulation aneurysms [1] and served well for some 30 years. It was a more precise and limited opening than the formerly used generous frontotemporal craniotomy. The success of the pterional craniotomy would not have been possible without the simultaneous introduction of the surgical microscope.

The advent of endovascular techniques, however, called for less invasive surgical procedures, as patients with the choice of less traumatic alternatives no longer accepted the traditional "big" openings. Further reduction of the craniotomy size was only possible by giving up the concept of one standard craniotomy for the principal anterior circulation aneurysms. Smaller craniotomies must be placed optimally and centered on the most direct path to the neck of the aneurysm. Moreover, the approach needs to allow safe control of the parent arteries. Although the exposure of the aneurysm and the parent arteries should be done in a manner that is focused on the pathology, safety and control are the principal rules for aneurysm surgery. Minimally invasive approaches must never be narrow and confining. Otherwise, disaster in the event of intraoperative aneurysm rupture is unavoidable. Minimizing the craniotomy potentially may compromise safety by reducing control of the parent artery, by limiting the view of perforating branches, and by restricting the degrees of freedom for surgical manipulation. This potential conflict must be kept in mind, as the safety of the procedure must be seen as the first priority. In our experience, a diameter of less than 4 cm is too small for general application, though smaller craniotomies can be considered exceptionally for certain unruptured aneurysms.

Prior to surgery, a master plan of the craniotomy and the approach to the aneurysm should be made, identifying the most direct route to the aneurysm that requires minimal retraction and minimal microsurgical dissection. In our experience, it is important to discriminate between aneurysms accessible through basal approaches (e.g., aneurysms of the carotid artery) and aneurysms accessible through hemispheric approaches (e.g., middle cerebral artery [MCA] and pericallosal artery aneurysms). The orientation and the exact placement of a small craniotomy for aneurysms reachable through approaches near the skull base are facilitated by the presence of enough anatomical landmarks, whereas a hemispheric approach is better performed with the help of navigation.

We use four different tailored craniotomies for the aneurysms of the anterior circle of Willis

H.-J. Steiger et al., *Microsurgical Brain Aneurysms: Illustrated Concepts and Cases*,
DOI 10.1007/978-3-662-45679-8_4, © Springer-Verlag Berlin Heidelberg 2015

(Fig. 4.1): the orbitocraniotomy for aneurysms of the anterior communicating artery, the pterional craniotomy for aneurysms of the internal carotid artery, the Sylvian craniotomy for the MCA aneurysm, and a small interhemispheric craniotomy for distal aneurysms of the anterior cerebral artery (i.e., at the origin of the callosomarginal artery). For aneurysms of the posterior circulation that are addressed by microsurgery (i.e., vertebral artery–posterior inferior cerebellar artery (PICA) aneurysms and peripheral aneurysms of the cerebellar arteries), either a lateral paracondylar targeted craniotomy or a paramedian opening is used.

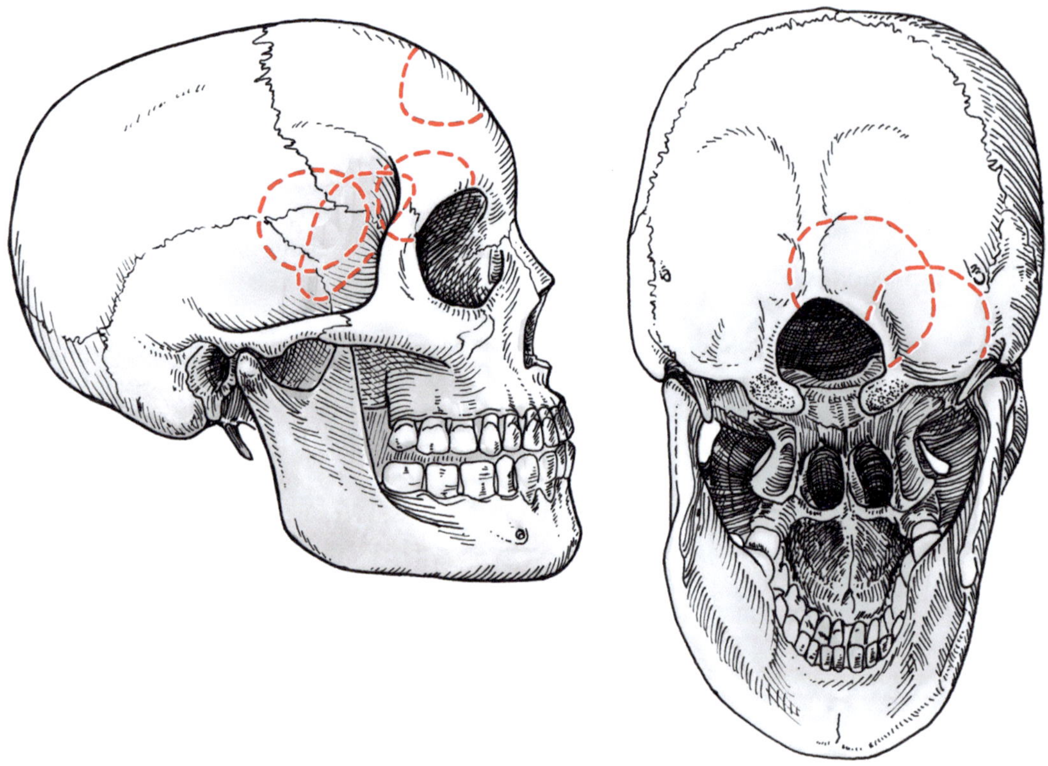

Fig. 4.1 Four different tailored craniotomies are used for typical anterior circulation aneurysms: pterional craniotomy for internal carotid aneurysms, Sylvian craniotomy for middle cerebral aneurysms, orbitocraniotomy for anterior communicating artery, and anterior interhemispheric craniotomy for A2-callosomarginal artery aneurysms. Two approaches are used for posterior circulation aneurysms: lateral paracondylar for vertebral artery aneurysms and paramedian for peripheral aneurysms

4.1.2 CSF Drainage

Brain retraction should be avoided as far as possible. Brain relaxation is achieved by cisternal, ventricular, or spinal drainage of cerebrospinal fluid (CSF) and by administering mannitol, if necessary. We use a spinal or ventricular catheter for all aneurysm operations in the acute stage after subarachnoid hemorrhage (Fig. 4.2). Lumbar spinal drainage is preferred for good-grade patients (World Federation of Neurosurgical Societies [WFNS] I or II), and ventricular drainage is preferred for WFNS grades III to V. In these latter patients, the ventricular catheter is routinely inserted at the time of admission via a frontal burr hole at Kocher's point. In order to avoid stress, this procedure is done under general anesthesia and the patient remains deeply sedated and intubated until the aneurysm has been secured surgically or by endovascular coiling.

Space-occupying hematomas are an exception; initial ventricular drainage is contraindicated for these patients because of the time lost and the substantial risk of rerupture. Efficient craniotomy and evacuation of the hematoma is the quickest and most efficient way to decrease intracranial pressure in these cases.

In good-grade patients, the lumbar catheter is inserted after induction of general anesthesia for the aneurysm procedure and removed at the end of the procedure.

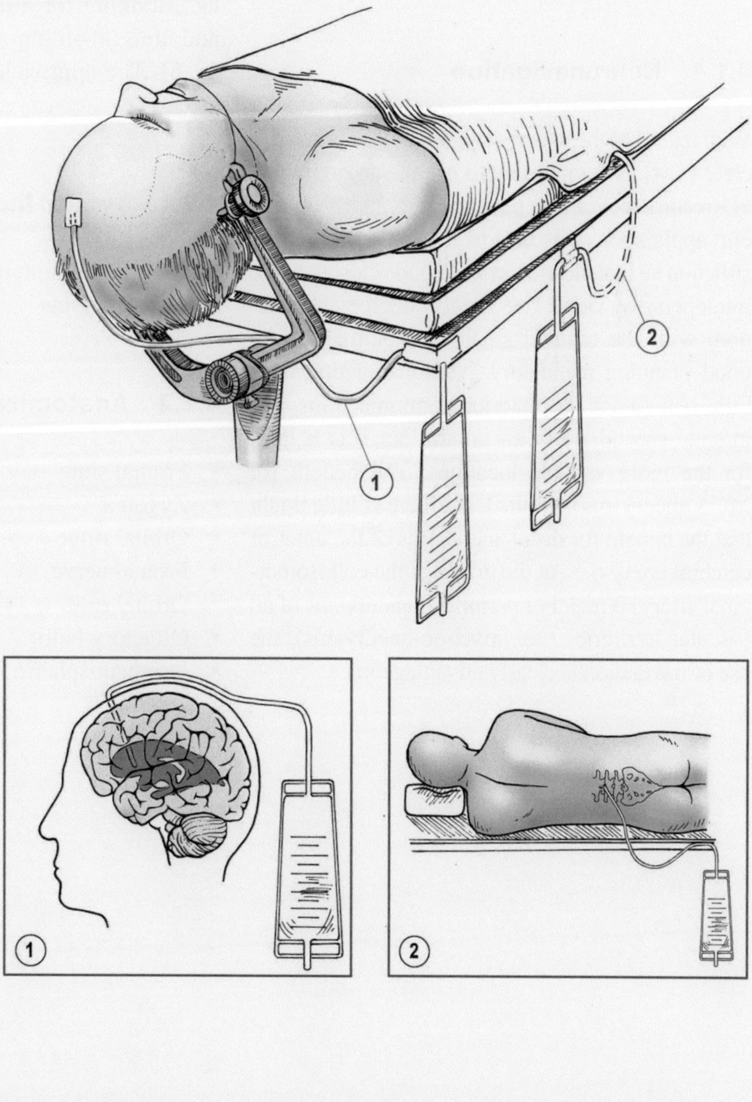

Fig. 4.2 Either ventricular (1) or spinal (2) cerebrospinal fluid (CSF) drainage is used for all patients with ruptured aneurysms

4.1.3 Intraoperative Monitoring

In contrast to brain tumor surgery, electrophysiological monitoring and navigation have not been generally accepted for aneurysm surgery. The reasons are explained by the nonelective nature of most aneurysm procedures. Electrophysiological monitoring cannot prevent all ischemic complications. For example, when losing a parent artery or perforating branch, the warning signs from monitoring are of little consequence. On the other hand, electrophysiological monitoring can recognize the inadvertent occlusion of an arterial branch [2]. In this situation, revision of clip positions may solve the problem and prevent permanent damage, so we recommend inclusion of electrophysiological monitoring whenever possible.

4.1.4 Neuronavigation

With regard to the use of navigation, things are less clear [3, 4]. It is important to use the angiographic 3D reconstruction for planning the approach and clip application. It is best to rotate the 3D reconstruction so that the view corresponds closely to the intraoperative view. The limited degrees of freedom with the tailored small craniotomies make good planning mandatory. Neuronavigation adds little benefit for the anterior communicating and internal carotid artery aneurysm, but it is helpful for the more variable locations. The benefit for MCA aneurysms is limited, but there is little doubt that the benefit for distal aneurysms of the anterior cerebral artery (i.e., at the origin of the callosomarginal artery) is real. For peripheral aneurysms of all vascular territories (i.e., mycotic aneurysms), the use of navigation is clearly advantageous.

4.1.5 Positioning

Surgical positioning deserves a great degree of attention and needs to be seen mainly in the context of approach planning. General principles to prevent pressure lesions and cranial venous stasis clearly need to be respected, but positioning also needs to be ergonomically optimized to allow the surgeon to work in a natural posture.

4.2 Orbitocraniotomy for Anterior Communicating Artery Aneurysms

We introduced orbitocraniotomy as the standard surgical approach for anterior communicating artery aneurysms some two decades ago, looking for a more ventral line of access and thus avoiding necessary brain retraction [5, 6]. The approach has proved to be safe and effective.

4.2.1 Typical Indications

- Anterior communicating artery aneurysms
- A1 aneurysms

4.2.2 Anatomical Landmarks

- Frontal sinus
- Zygoma
- Orbital ridge
- Frontal nerve
- Orbital roof
- Olfactory bulb
- Interhemispheric fissure

4.2.3 Positioning and Skin Incision

After induction of endotracheal anesthesia, a spinal drainage catheter is inserted in all good-grade patients operated on acutely after subarachnoid hemorrhage. Ventriculostomy is inserted at the time of admission in patients admitted in WFNS grade IV or V.

The patients are placed in a supine position with the head rotated 45° to the side opposite the planned craniotomy (Fig. 4.3). All anterior communicating artery aneurysms are approached principally from the side of the dominant A1 segment. Approaching from the side of the dominant A1 segment allows for control of the aneurysm with minimal dissection and manipulation of adjacent cerebral structures. The 45° initial rotation represents an average starting point. Occasionally, a more lateral or a more anterior view is necessary during surgery. Fine adjustments of the head rotation during surgery are accomplished by tilting the operating table. The neck of the patient is moderately hyperextended, resulting in an angle of 10–20° between the plane of the anterior cranial fossa and the vertical plane. This position allows the orbital cortex to fall away from the orbital roof, thus minimizing the need for brain retraction. With 45° of head rotation, it is generally not necessary to use a cushion to support the ipsilateral shoulder. A shoulder support may be required in selected patients with degenerative changes of the cervical spine and consequent limited range of motion.

The head is secured in a Mayfield clamp, with the clamp positioned as horizontally as possible. During adjustment and balancing of the surgical microscope, care should be taken that the neutral baseline position of the objective tube is set at an angle 20° from vertical. This position allows easy manipulation of the microscope within the entire range of motion necessary for the orbitocranial approach.

We recommend a temporofrontal hairline skin incision, although an eyebrow incision is a viable alternative. The skin incision is started 1 cm in front of the tragus and slightly above the zygomatic arch. After a cautious incision has been made in the skin and the galea, the superficial temporal artery within the temporal fascia is identified. The frontal or parietal branch of the artery is divided if necessary, and a small hemoclip is used to secure the proximal stump. The scalp incision is extended to the frontal midline.

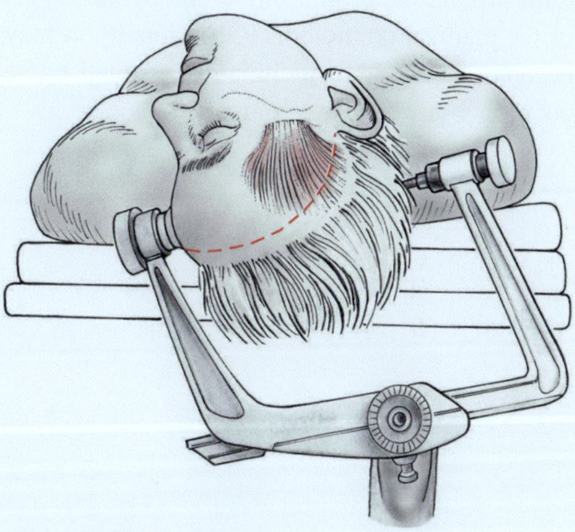

Fig. 4.3 Positioning with the head rotated some 45° and moderately hyperextended

4.2.4 Soft Tissue Dissection

The skin flap is gently elevated and turned back. Dissection is performed in the interfascial plane between the temporal fascia and the aponeurosis of the temporal muscle. The supraorbital fat pad must be mobilized together with the scalp flap to prevent injury to the frontal branch of the facial nerve. The anterior attachment of the temporal muscle at the orbital pillar and the anterior aspect of the linea temporalis are incised sharply. The temporal muscle is then dissected from the underlying bone and pulled back using a galea hook (Fig. 4.4). The temporal muscle should not be mobilized more than absolutely necessary for the limited craniotomy. The lateral and superior orbital rims are then dissected from the periorbita using a blunt curved dissector. At this stage, attention should be paid to the frontal nerve as it turns around the orbital rim at the medial aspect of the planned craniotomy. Occasionally, it may become necessary to mobilize the frontal nerve out of its bony groove or tunnel.

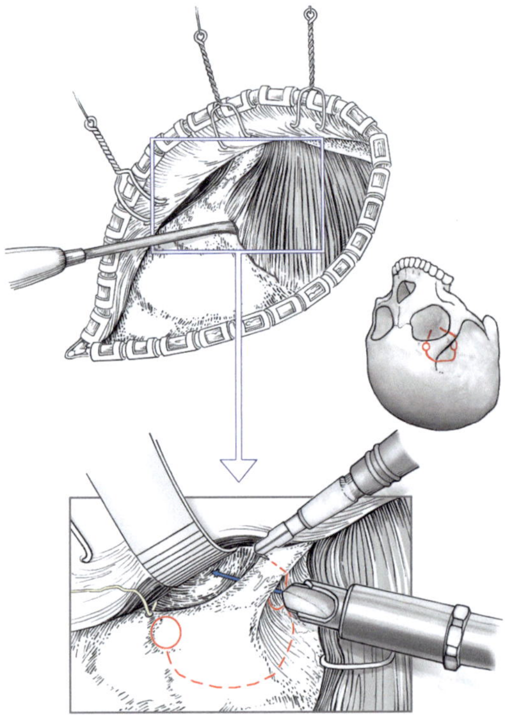

Fig. 4.4 Detachment of the anterior temporal muscle. Outline of orbitocraniotomy, which starts from two burr holes. The lateral burr hole is placed at the orbitozygomatic junction as the keyhole for the pterional craniotomy. In contrast to the pterional craniotomy, the axis of the burr is pointed more toward the orbit, so that the anterior cranial fossa and the orbit are opened simultaneously

4.2.5 Orbitocraniotomy

We use two burr holes for the craniotomy. The initial burr hole corresponds to the keyhole of the pterional craniotomy placed at the frontozygomatic suture. The direction of the burr hole, however, aims more toward the orbit so that the orbit and the anterior cranial fossa can be opened with this single burr hole (see Fig. 4.4). A second burr hole is then placed above the upper orbital rim at the medial aspect of the planned craniotomy. The dura is separated from the orbital roof and the convexity with the use of a blunt dissector. The two burr holes are then connected along the planned upper delineation of the orbitocraniotomy by using the craniotome (Fig. 4.5). A small bone saw is used to cut the superior and lateral orbital rims. The dura and the periorbita must be protected with a small spatula. The bone cut in the lateral orbital rim is extended down to the lateral burr hole. At the medial burr hole, the orbital roof must be cut as far down as possible. The posterior aspect of the medial orbital roof is divided through the medial burr hole with a small punch or a diamond drill. At the lateral burr hole, the orbital roof is divided along the pterion to a depth of 3–4 cm with the use of a small punch. The bone flap is then elevated, and the orbital roof is fractured between the end of the medial and lateral orbital roof incisions. Care should be taken to place the fracture line as far back as possible. We do not advocate removal of the residual orbital roof in an osteoclastic manner after the bone flap is turned. In that event, the orbital roof must be reconstructed later with foreign material to prevent orbital roof instability with enophthalmos or pulsating exophthalmos.

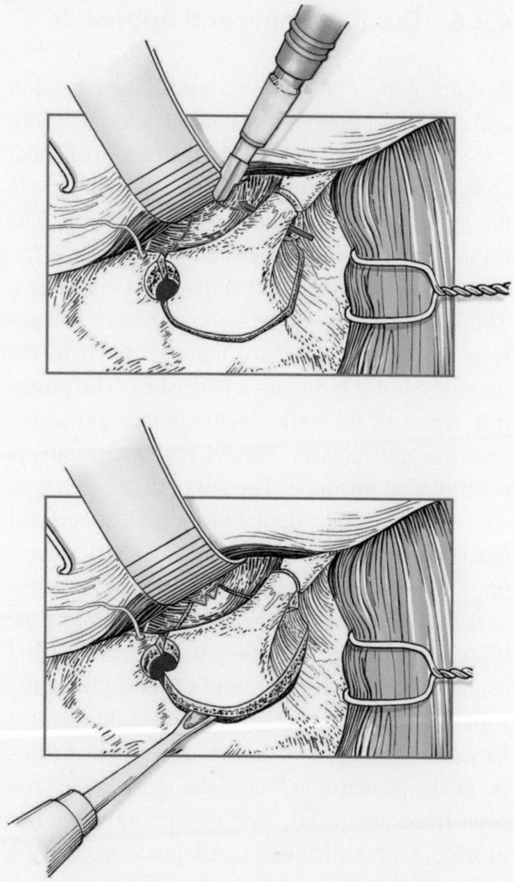

Fig. 4.5 The burr holes are then connected through the frontal bone by using a craniotome. The medial and lateral orbital rims are cut with a small blade saw. The lateral bone cut is extended down to the lateral burr hole. The lateral and medial aspects of the orbital roof are divided through the burr holes with the blade saw or a punch. The bone flap is then elevated, and the orbital roof is fractured as far toward the apex of the orbit as possible

4.2.6 Dural Opening and Approach

A dural flap is created in a curvilinear fashion and reflected basally. The dural incision does not cross the Sylvian fissure. After the dura is opened, approximately 50–100 mL of CSF is drained via the spinal drainage or the ventriculostomy. The orbital cortex is gently elevated. At this stage, the central aspect of the Sylvian fissure is visualized. This central aspect of the Sylvian fissure is carefully split in the ordinary manner down to the internal carotid bifurcation (Fig. 4.6). The posterior aspect of the gyrus rectus is then separated from the optic chiasm. The A1 segment usually is controlled at this time. The next critical step is to split the interhemispheric fissure. The superficial arachnoid layer is opened by using a small microhook. The interhemispheric arachnoid adhesions in the deeper layers can be separated by using the bipolar forceps in a spreading motion such as that usually performed at the level of the Sylvian fissure. The projection of the aneurysm dome must be taken into account during this stage. At this point, the posterior aspect of the gyrus rectus has been freed completely and can be mobilized to provide access to the A1–A2 junction and the anterior communicating artery. The exposure is stabilized by using a small spatula. To prevent damage to the orbital cortex, the brain is supported at the lateral and medial border of the craniotomy with a rolled cotton pledget to distribute the pressure on the frontal cortex. Occasionally, the projection of the aneurysm fundus renders formal splitting of the interhemispheric fissure inappropriate. In this situation, a small medial reduction of the gyrus rectus must be performed. However, it is always possible to limit the resection to the portion of the gyrus rectus medial to the olfactory tract.

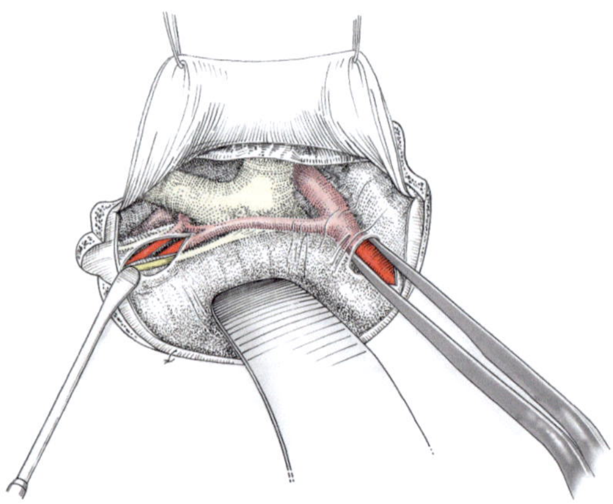

Fig. 4.6 Following dural opening, the central aspect of the Sylvian fissure is opened, as well as the suprachiasmatic cistern and the interhemispheric fissure

4.2.7 Closure

The dura is closed in standard watertight fashion. The periorbita is injured occasionally during dissection from the orbital roof. To prevent protrusion of the orbital fat, periorbital tears should be repaired immediately with a suture. If the frontal sinus has been opened at the medial aspect of the opening, the defect is plugged with a muscle graft taken from the temporalis muscle. We do not recommend use of a pediculated periosteal flap with the orbitocraniotomy, because it risks interference with eyelid and eyebrow motility. The bone flap is repositioned and attached by using small titanium platelets. The anterior aspect of the temporalis muscle is reattached at the linea temporalis. For this purpose, two tangential burr holes are made in the bone flap, and the muscle is reattached with two 3–0 sutures.

4.2.8 Pitfalls and Complications

- Dural and periorbital laceration
- Frontal nerve injuries
- CSF fistula due to insufficient plugging of the frontal sinus and dural closure
- Pressure injuries to orbital contents

4.3 Frontal Interhemispheric Approach to Pericallosal Artery Aneurysms

There are two different variants in this access, supranasal and high frontal. Supranasal access is used for aneurysms close to the genu of the corpus callosum, whereas high frontal access is used for supracallosal locations [7]. As with all interhemispheric approaches, it is necessary to avoid retraction injury during access. Therefore, we recommend lumbar or ventricular CSF drainage for all aneurysms, including unruptured ones.

Because the location of pericallosal artery aneurysms is quite variable, the use of image-guided neuronavigation is helpful and is therefore generally recommended for these aneurysms.

Most pericallosal artery aneurysms can be approached from either side. We recommend choosing the side that allows access to the aneurysm base and parent artery while avoiding the dome of the aneurysm. In patients with intracerebral hemorrhage, we recommend the approach on the side of the hemorrhage.

4.3.1 Typical Indications

- Pericallosal artery aneurysms
- Peripheral anterior cerebral artery aneurysms

4.3.2 Anatomical Landmarks

- Frontal sinus
- Coronal suture
- Superior sagittal sinus
- Parasagittal bridging veins
- Falx cerebri
- Cingulate gyrus
- Pericallosal artery
- Callosomarginal artery
- Crista galli

4.3.3 Positioning and Skin Incision

A flat supine position, with the patient looking straight up, is used for supranasal access. In contrast, for the high frontal access variant, the head is slightly inclined.

For the supranasal variant, a bicoronal incision in the hairline is created (Fig. 4.7). The skin, galea, and periosteum are reflected together. The temporal muscles remain untouched. It is usually not necessary to extend the skin incision laterally down to the zygoma, but just enough to enable reflection of the skin flap to free the planned craniotomy.

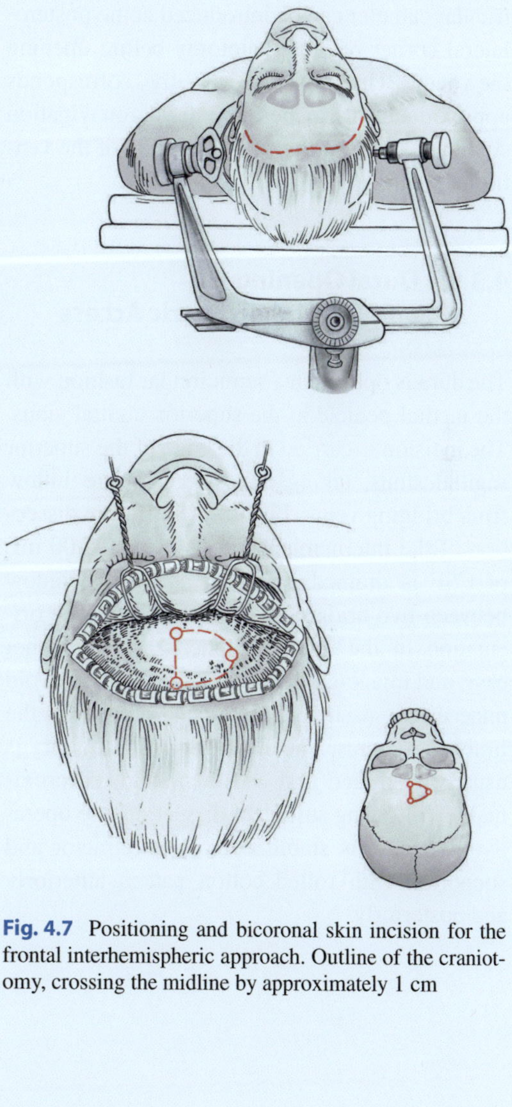

Fig. 4.7 Positioning and bicoronal skin incision for the frontal interhemispheric approach. Outline of the craniotomy, crossing the midline by approximately 1 cm

4.3.4 Craniotomy and Ventricular Drainage

A triangular or rectangular 4×4 cm craniotomy extending 1 cm across the midline is recommended (see Fig. 4.7). A smaller craniotomy limits the opportunity to find a suitable access between the bridging veins. The basal variant craniotomy is placed immediately above the frontal sinus. It is particularly important to ensure that the frontal sinus is not opened unnoticed by basal placement of burr holes for dural tacking sutures.

If no working CSF drainage is in place, a ventricular catheter can be introduced at the posterolateral corner of the craniotomy before opening the dura. This location usually corresponds approximately to Kocher's point. Neuronavigation should be used for the exact direction of the ventricular catheter.

4.3.5 Dural Opening and Interhemispheric Access

The dura is opened in a semicircular fashion with the medial pedicle at the superior sagittal sinus. The incision is carried to the edge of the superior sagittal sinus, taking care not to injure inflow from bridging veins (Fig. 4.8) [8]. Before dissection of the interhemispheric fissure, 50–100 mL of CSF is drained. First, an adequate window between two bridging veins is selected. The orientation in the interhemispheric fissure is not easy, and image-guided orientation helps to avoid unnecessary tissue dissection and damage to the limbic structures. The distal pericallosal artery is usually identified first and then followed proximally. Following sufficient dissection, the operative exposure is stabilized with a retractor and supported with rolled cotton patties anteriorly and posteriorly.

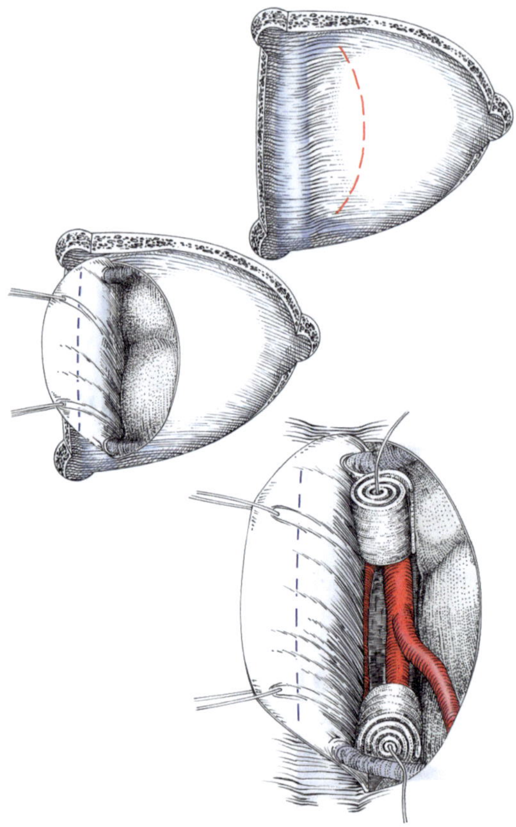

Fig. 4.8 Dural opening, taking care not to injure bridging veins. Dissection of the interhemispheric fissure and visualization of the pericallosal artery

4.3.6 Wound Closure

The dura is closed in the usual way. If the tip of the frontal sinus is opened, it is sealed with a muscle plug or similar.

4.3.7 Pitfalls and Complications

- CSF fistula through inadvertently opened frontal sinus
- Hemorrhagic infarction due to retraction and venous injury
- Dissection damage to the limbic system caused by disorientation

4.4 Keyhole Approach to Middle Cerebral Artery Aneurysms (Sylvian Craniotomy)

Many approaches have been described for MCA aneurysms. They vary by their skin and muscle incisions and the placement of the bone opening. The craniotomies for MCA aneurysms can be divided into frontolateral and temporal approaches. Many authors prefer to approach the aneurysm by following the proximal MCA (M1) from the internal carotid artery (ICA) bifurcation. Others prefer to approach the MCA bifurcation inward from the Sylvian fissure or through the superior temporal gyrus. At first sight, controlling M1 from the ICA bifurcation appears to be a matter of safety. In reality, however, accessing M1 close to the ICA bifurcation requires considerable retraction onto the fronto-orbital cortex, as well as maneuvering around the aneurysm. It is important to note that (particularly in cases of an elongated M1) this artery runs high in its middle segment before turning downward again at the bifurcation. We prefer to control M1 from the periphery. M1 is identified by following the superior trunks (M2) of the MCA proximally. Depending on the exact anatomy of the bifurcation and the aneurysm, M1 is controlled either between the MCA main branches or on the frontal side of the superior M2 trunk. A limited Sylvian craniotomy usually serves well for the typical MCA aneurysm [9]. Neuronavigation can be helpful but cannot be considered mandatory [3].

4.4.1 Typical Indications

- MCA main bifurcation aneurysms
- Peripheral MCA aneurysms

4.4.2 Anatomical Landmarks

- Superficial temporal artery
- Frontozygomatic point
- Sylvian line
- Pterion
- Middle meningeal artery

4.4.3 Positioning and Skin Incision

For the normal approach to MCA aneurysms, the head is positioned with a 45° rotation to the contralateral side (Fig. 4.9). Three main landmarks should be identified on the scalp before application of the surgical drapes: the frontozygomatic point, the Sylvian line, and the pterion. The frontozygomatic point is located on the orbital rim 2.5 cm above the level at which the upper edge of the zygomatic arch joins the orbital rim and just below the junction of the lateral and superior aspects of the orbital rim. The Sylvian fissure is located along a line that extends backward from the frontozygomatic point across the lateral surface of the head to the three-quarter point, 75 % of the distance between the nasion and the inion on the midline. The pterion, which represents the site on the external surface of the cranium approximating the lateral end of the sphenoid ridge, is located 2–3 cm behind the frontozygomatic point, on the path of the Sylvian fissure line. Even when this area shows anatomic variations from one individual to another, there is a bony depression following the main axis of the Sylvian line. This depression is easily detected beneath the temporal muscle by firm palpation over the temporal area.

A limited hairline incision is fashioned that allows sufficient exposure down to the orbital rim. The temporal muscle is incised, and the anterior portion of the muscle is mobilized together with the skin flap.

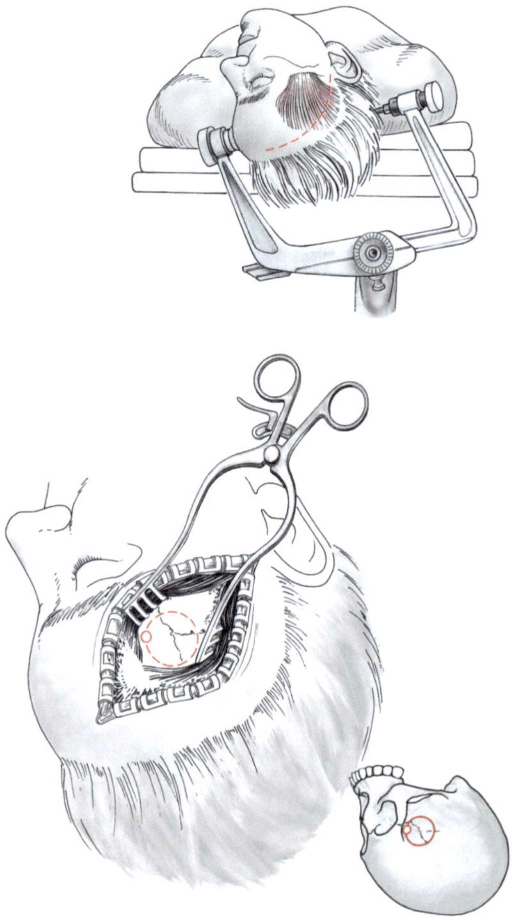

Fig. 4.9 Positioning and limited frontotemporal skin incision. Outline of the craniotomy. Two thirds should be placed above the Sylvian groove and one third below

4.4.4 Craniotomy

A round craniotomy 3–4 cm in diameter is well suited for adequate control and clipping of MCA aneurysms. The craniotomy should be placed on the Sylvian fissure, immediately behind the orbital rim. Two thirds of the craniotomy should lie above the Sylvian fissure and one third below (see Fig. 4.9). The craniotomy is usually above the sphenoid ridge, but occasionally, a large sphenoid ridge may block inferior cutting with the craniotome, necessitating the use of a diamond drill.

4.4.5 Dural Opening and Opening the Sylvian Fissure

It is best to open the dura in a Y-shaped fashion (Fig. 4.10). The Sylvian vein is identified. Adequate brain relaxation must be achieved now by draining 50–100 mL of CSF. In case of subarachnoid hemorrhage, we recommend a lumbar or ventricular catheter. If relaxation is insufficient, mannitol (1–2 g/kg of body weight) is also given. Only in the situation of a major intracerebral hematoma is sufficient relaxation achieved solely by the evacuation of the hematoma. The Sylvian fissure is subsequently split on the frontal side of the Sylvian vein. One to three venous branches crossing the fissure usually must be coagulated and divided. It is important to split the Sylvian fissure all the way down to the sphenoid ridge to allow for separation of the frontal and temporal lobes. Sufficient dissection at this stage avoids the need for excessive retraction on the frontal operculum. The superior trunk of the MCA is then identified in the depth of the Sylvian fissure (Fig. 4.11). This artery is subsequently followed proximally to the MCA bifurcation.

To secure proximal control, it is important to have the course of M1 and the projection of the aneurysm in mind. Most MCA aneurysms are directed more or less toward the temporal lobe, but some are attached to the frontal side. Therefore,

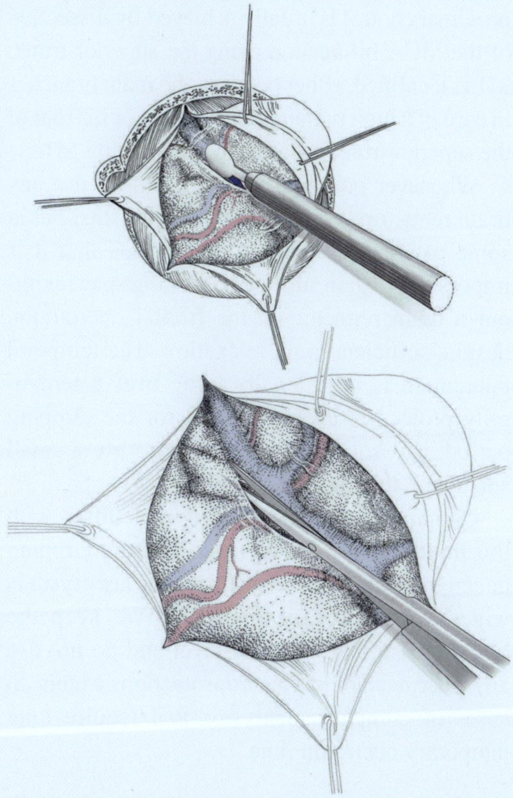

Fig. 4.10 Dural opening in a Y-shaped fashion. The Sylvian fissure is usually opened above the Sylvian vein

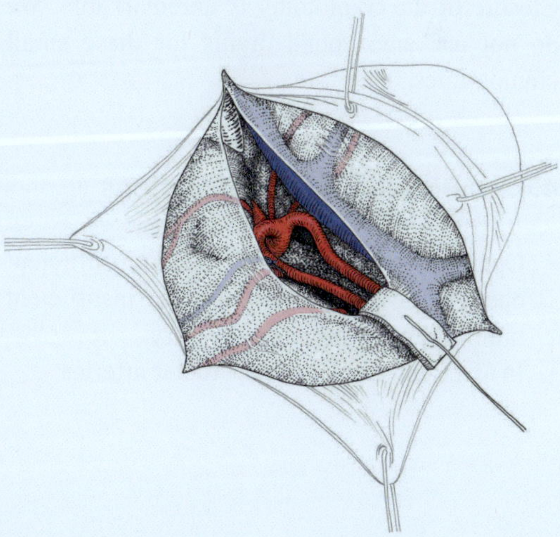

Fig. 4.11 Dissection of the Sylvian fissure and visualization of the M2 segments

proximal control is usually achieved by dissection of the MCA bifurcation along the superior trunk. M1 is identified, either between the main branches in case of a high running M1 segment or in front of the superior trunk in case of a low running M1.

Whenever possible, we prefer not to use any brain retractors at all for MCA aneurysms, but in some patients, the brain is so swollen that it is impossible to gain sufficient working space without a brain retractor on the frontal operculum, despite sufficient brain relaxation. The temporal operculum is occasionally lying over a temporally projecting aneurysm, and for the clipping period, it is sometimes necessary to use a small spatula on the temporal operculum.

Clipping the aneurysm does not differ with this limited approach. We use temporary clipping generously whenever the neck of the aneurysm is wider than the diameter of M1. We keep the blood pressure at a normal level and do not use any pharmacological neuroprotection, except in cases of complex aneurysms that require long temporary occlusion time.

4.4.6 Wound Closure

Closure of the craniotomy is unremarkable. We do not use any wound drains for these small craniotomies.

4.4.7 Pitfalls and Complications

- Opercular retraction injury due to insufficient opening of the Sylvian fissure, insufficient brain relaxation, or venous injury
- Inadvertent sacrifice of opercular arteries

4.5 Pterional Approach to Internal Carotid Artery Aneurysms

This approach was formally developed by Yasargil et al. [10], and several authors contributed to perfecting the technique [11–13]. The following is a detailed description of a standardized procedure from among the multiple versions that has proven advantageous.

4.5.1 Typical Indications

- Aneurysms of the internal carotid artery
- Alternative approach for aneurysms of the anterior cerebral artery (A1 and anterior communicating artery)
- Aneurysms of the proximal MCA

4.5.2 Anatomical Landmarks

- Temporal fascia
- Superficial temporal artery
- Temporal muscle
- Zygomatic branches of the facial nerve
- Orbital ridge
- Sphenoid bone (small and large sphenoid wing)
- Zygomatic process of the frontal bone
- Pterion
- Middle meningeal artery
- Sylvian vein
- Anterior clinoid process

4.5.3 Positioning and Skin Incision

The patient is supine, with the head rotated 45° to the opposite side. Support of the ipsilateral shoulder is not necessary for patients with a normally mobile cervical spine. The Mayfield clamp is placed horizontally. The singular Mayfield pin should be centered above the mastoid behind the ear on the side of the craniotomy. The paired pins are inserted contralaterally above the ear and above the temporal line (i.e., located outside the temporal muscle).

In addition to the rotation of 45° to the opposite side, the head is slightly lifted and reclined 10–15°, so that the brain spontaneously falls back from the base of the skull, thus minimizing the need for retraction (Fig. 4.12). The central reference point for the craniotomy is the frontozygomatic articulation (keyhole). The degree to which the head is reclined can be optimized individually for the specific location of the aneurysm. The same applies to the head rotation to the opposite side. The standard rotation of 45° is a mean value, which can also be modified or customized intraoperatively by rotation of the operating table.

As with any patient position, the cooperation of the anesthesiologist is mandatory; the uninhibited freedom of venous reflux and ventilation must be verified before covering the patient.

The arc-shaped skin incision begins at the zygoma in front of the ear. The distance to the tragus should be only 5 mm, in order to avoid infringing on the frontal branch of the facial nerve. To prevent inadvertent division of the main trunk of the superficial temporal artery, it is best identified and marked before skin incision, but it is usually necessary to divide either the frontal or the parietal branch of this artery. The proximal stump should be carefully coagulated or occluded with a small hemoclip, as this artery has a tendency to open, leading to postoperative subcutaneous hemorrhage. The scalp incision then follows approximately the normal hairline to the frontal midline.

The scalp should not be separated from the temporal muscle more than necessary. The muscle is divided here according to the posterior limit of the planned craniotomy. In addition, the muscle insertion at the temporal line should be cut and not be stripped off the bone, leaving a strip of the fascia for later anchoring of the muscle. The muscle is then separated from the bone down to the orbital ridge. The orbital rim should not be exceeded during dissection with a periosteal elevator, as doing so usually leads to a postoperative monocular hematoma. The muscle and skin are then retracted with the help of galea hooks.

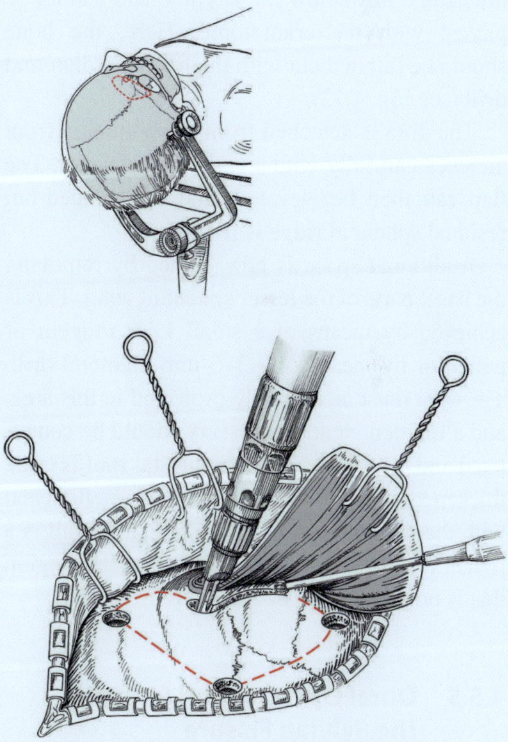

Fig. 4.12 Positioning and outline of the pterional craniotomy. Bone cutting with a craniotome and ball drill for the basal sphenoid ridge

4.5.4 Craniotomy

Our standard procedure uses four holes to minimize the chance of dural laceration. If the dura separates easily from the bone (particularly in younger patients), the craniotomy can be accomplished with only one or two burr holes. The first hole (keyhole) is created directly below the temporal line, immediately above the frontozygomatic suture. The drilling direction must point slightly upward in order to avoid penetration of the orbit. The craniotomy is then drawn anteriorly some 2 cm immediately above the orbital ridge, then upward to the temporal line, and finally to the squama temporalis above the zygomatic arch. On the inner bone surface, the sphenoid ridge lies below the keyhole and cannot be passed with the craniotome. Here, the bone should be thinned out with the help of a diamond drill (see Fig. 4.12).

The dura is detached from the bone flap from all sides carefully with a periosteal elevator. The flap can then be elevated, and the thinned-out residual sphenoid ridge is fractured.

Additional space is now gained by removing the basal parts of the lesser sphenoid wing. This is achieved by means of a small Luer rongeur or punch or by means of a 3–5-mm diamond drill. The dura must be carefully protected in this area, and a frequent venous emissary should be coagulated and cut. Sometimes, the orbital roof is quite thickened with bumps. These can also be flattened with the diamond drill, so that the end result is a pyramid-shaped access to the perisellar region that is not obstructed by any bony structures.

4.5.5 Dural Opening and Splitting the Sylvian Fissure

The dural opening is fashioned in an arcuate way, crossing the Sylvian fissure (Fig. 4.13). The Sylvian fissure is split in the lateral portion of the exposure on the frontal side of the Sylvian vein. The degree of necessary opening of the fissure depends on the specific case. Extensive splitting may not be necessary for a proximal ICA aneurysm. On the other hand, complete opening of the proximal fissure is mandatory for terminal aneurysms of the ICA. Complete opening of the Sylvian fissure mandates division of some frontal vein branches (Fig. 4.14).

A retractor (8–10 mm wide) can now be placed on the orbital cortex, and the basal cisterns can be opened (Fig. 4.15).

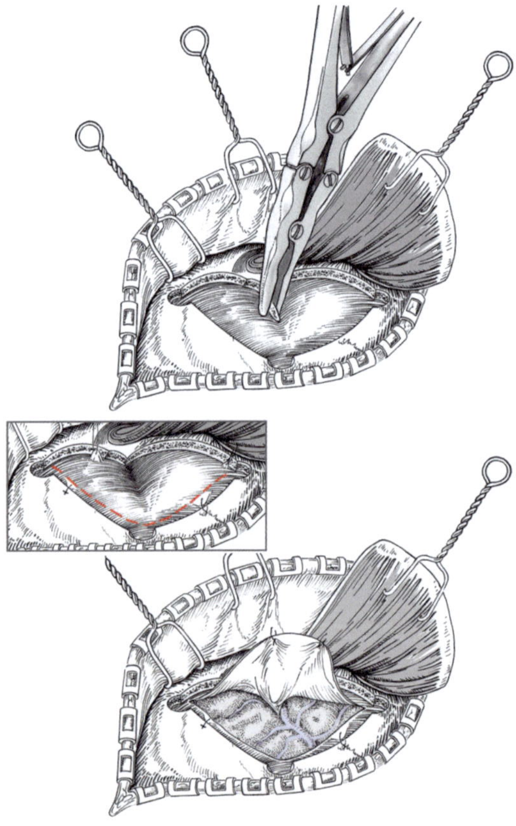

Fig. 4.13 Removal of residual pterion. Arcuate dural opening crossing the Sylvian fissure

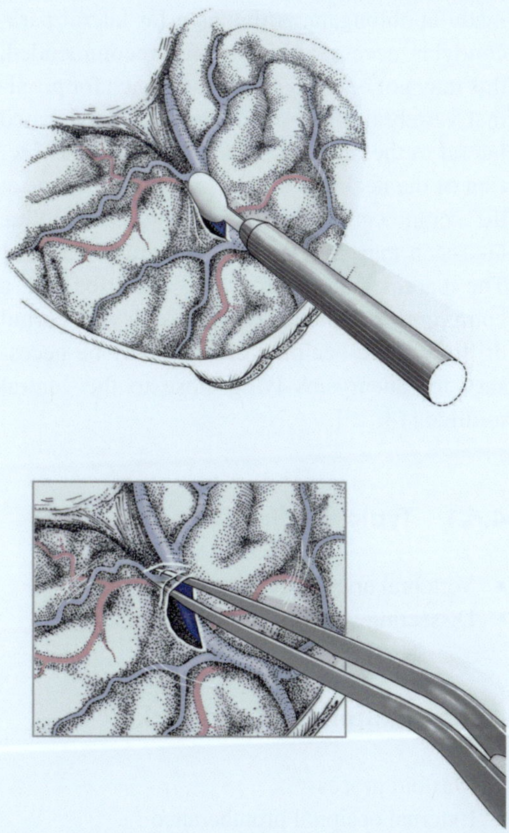

Fig. 4.14 Opening the Sylvian fissure, usually above the Sylvian vein. Frontal branches of the Sylvian vein must be coagulated and divided

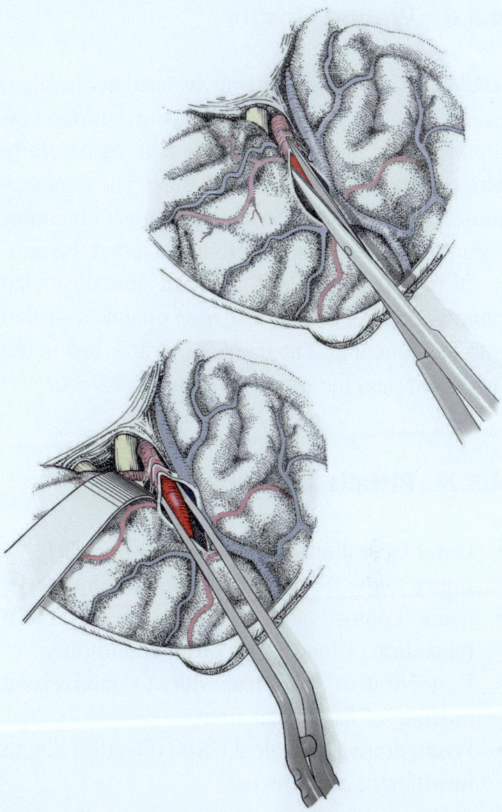

Fig. 4.15 Central opening of the fissure. Opening the basal cisterns

4.5.6 Wound Closure

The dura is closed in a watertight fashion. Sometimes, the frontal sinus is opened during craniotomy, and in this case, it needs to be carefully plugged and covered during closure. The temporal muscle is attached to the temporal line with nonresorbable sutures. If no soft tissue is left at the temporal line, the muscle is attached directly to the bone with the help of V-shaped channels drilled into the bone flap. The bone flap is attached in the usual way, and the wound is closed in layers.

4.5.7 Pitfalls and Complications

- Dural laceration, particularly in the elderly
- Injury to the frontal branch of the facial nerve
- Brain contusions due to insufficient brain relaxation or inadequate basal craniotomy
- Postoperative CSF leak due to inadvertent opening of the frontal sinus
- Postoperative subgaleal CSF collection due to insufficient dura closure

4.6 Paracondylar Approach to Vertebral Artery Aneurysms

When planning the approach to vertebral artery aneurysms, it is important to keep in mind the position of the aneurysm in relation to the medulla oblongata. Although a far lateral paracondylar access is commonly recommended, this may not be the optimum approach for proximal vertebral artery aneurysms that are located lateral to the medulla oblongata. The cross section of the neck has a transversely oval shape at the craniocervical junction, so a midline approach may provide a shorter line of access. The paramedian approach as described is a compromise. More lateral extension with partial drilling of the occipital condyle may be necessary for aneurysms lying close to the ventral midline [14, 15].

4.6.1 Typical Indications

- Vertebral artery–PICA aneurysm
- Dissecting vertebral artery aneurysm

4.6.2 Anatomical Landmarks

- Mastoid process
- External occipital protuberance
- Sternocleidomastoid muscle
- Occipital artery
- Asterion
- Posterior arc of atlas
- Occipital condyles
- Vertebral artery
- Sigmoid sinus
- Caudal cranial nerves

4.6.3 Positioning and Skin Incision

Although a semisitting or sitting position may have its virtues, the park bench position is now generally favored (Fig. 4.16). The shoulders should be rotated about 45° away from the surgeon in order to be out of the line of access, and the head should be inclined as much as possible. The Mayfield pins must be placed in a plane perpendicular to the planned line of access, and the paired pins should be placed on the downside of the head.

A linear, vertical incision line 8–10 cm long is fashioned some 3 cm behind the mastoid fossa. The upper end of the incision corresponds to the upper edge of the ear helix, and the lower end corresponds approximately to C3 (Fig. 4.17). The occipital artery must be coagulated and divided. The proximal stump should be secured with a hemoclip.

It is necessary to spare the artery during skin incision if an occipital artery-to-PICA bypass is a planned option for a complex aneurysm. The artery can be spared either by fashioning a hook-shaped skin incision or by identifying the course of the occipital artery via Doppler prior to skin incision and then cutting down on the artery and following it until sufficient length is provided.

The muscle layers are split vertically en bloc and pushed off the bone. Care must be taken not to injure the extracranial vertebral artery close to the foramen magnum. The vertebral artery is difficult to palpate and should be identified with the help of a Doppler device (see Fig. 4.17).

The situs is then fixed with an angled spreader inserted from the top and a facultative second straight one from the bottom.

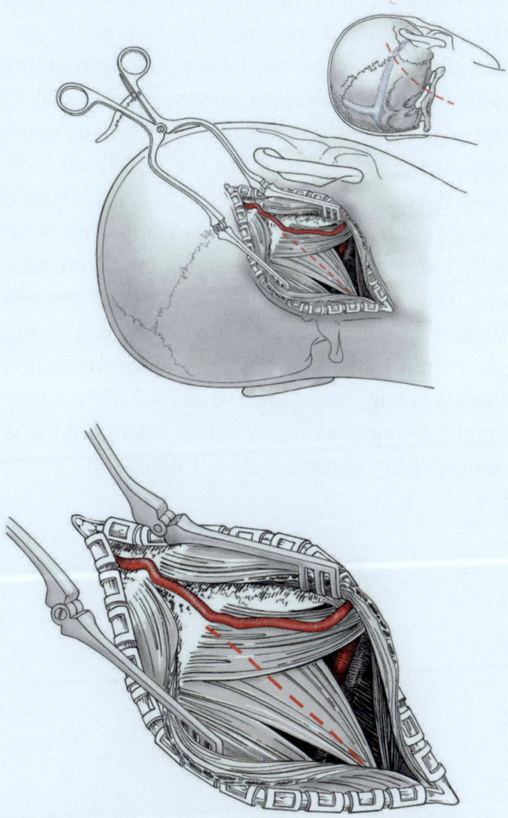

Fig. 4.17 Outline of the skin incision. Visualization of the occipital artery after splitting the splenius muscle. Splitting the deep muscular layer and identification of the vertebral artery

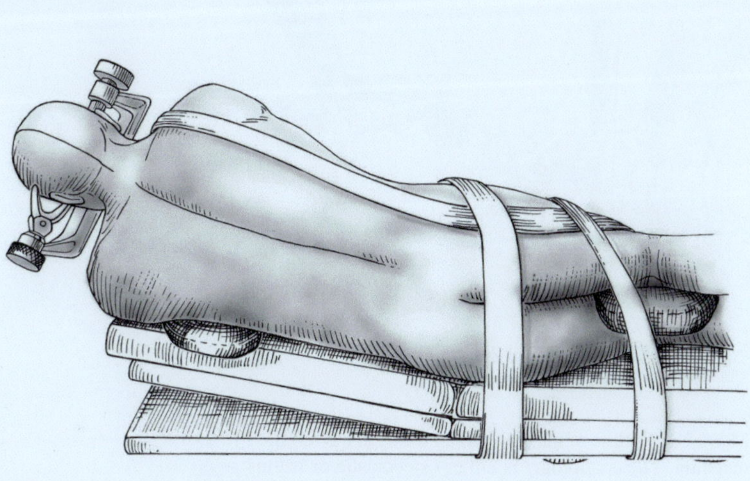

Fig. 4.16 Positioning in park bench configuration. The head may be slightly elevated to minimize venous congestion

4.6.4 Craniotomy

An osteoclastic craniotomy is preferred because even if a flap has been cut out first, substantial additional drilling laterally will be necessary (Fig. 4.18). The bone material is carefully preserved and may be used later in covering the defect. The opening is extended superolaterally to the edge of the sigmoid sinus. The venous emissary in the extension of the mastoid fossa indicates the location of the underlying sinus. Opened mastoid cells are sealed immediately with bone wax. Larger cells may require plugging with muscle. The craniotomy should measure at the end some 4 cm in diameter. Caudally, the craniotomy should reach the floor of the posterior fossa. It is usually not necessary to do work around the extracranial segment of the vertebral artery, and it is not necessary to remove the C1 hemiarch.

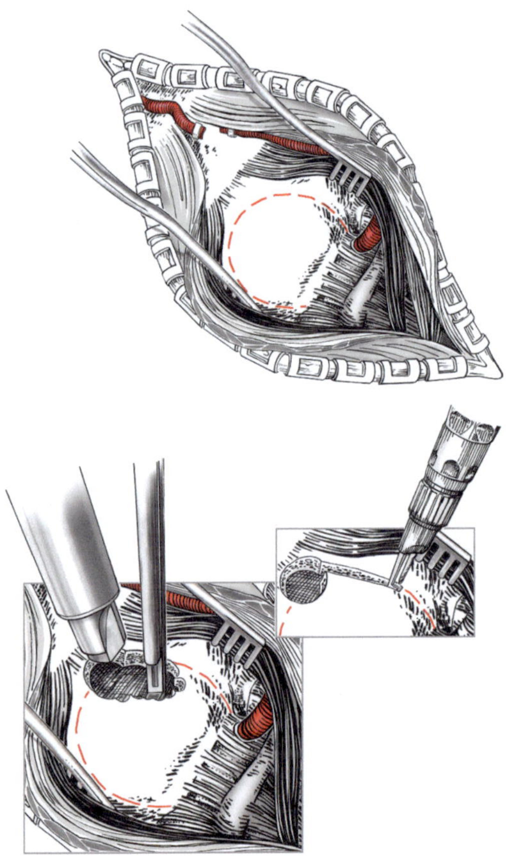

Fig. 4.18 Outline of the craniotomy down to the foramen magnum. The craniotomy is either osteoclastic or begins with removal of a bone flap

4.6.5 Dural Opening and Pontomedullary Dissection

The dura is opened in an arcuate fashion for exposure of the caudal cerebellopontine angle, caudally ending close to the midline (Fig. 4.19). CSF is drained primarily from the cisterna magna in order to relax conditions. Next, the cerebellum is carefully lifted with a retractor, and the cranial nerves IX to XI are identified.

The vertebral artery is then identified rostral to the dentate ligament. The origin of the PICA is usually located between the fascicles of the cranial nerves IX through XII, but it varies greatly (Fig. 4.20), and this factor is predominantly responsible for the risk of cranial nerve injury associated with the clipping of vertebral artery–PICA aneurysms.

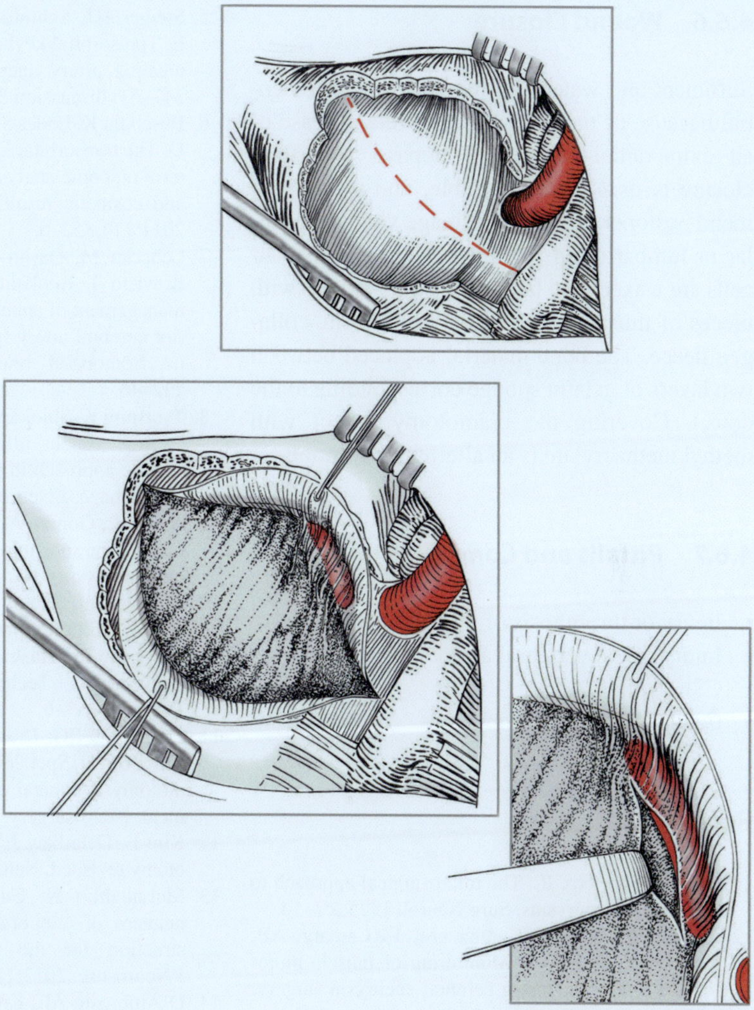

Fig. 4.19 Arcuate dural opening. Opening the basal cisterns and identification of the proximal intracranial vertebral artery

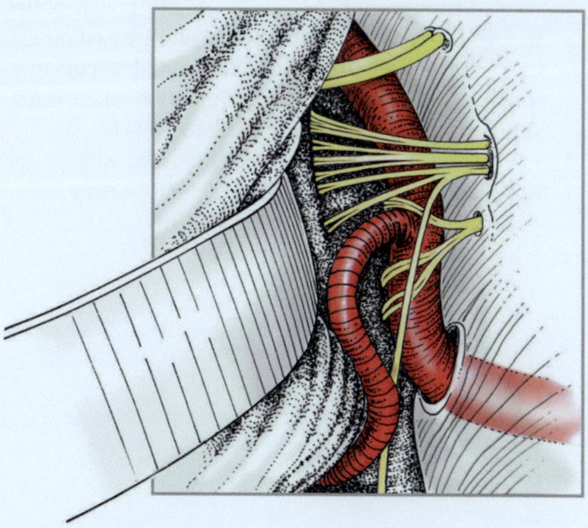

Fig. 4.20 Identification of caudal cranial nerves and the PICA origin

4.6.6 Wound Closure

Sufficient and watertight dural closure is essential because of the risk of CSF fistula. In case of an extracranial–intracranial bypass, watertight closure is usually not possible, and we recommend postoperative CSF drainage via a ventricular or lumbar drain for 5 days. The mastoid air cells are waxed, and larger cells are plugged with pieces of muscle and covered with fibrin–collagen fleece. The bone material is placed between two layers of gelatin sponge corresponding to the defect. Covering the craniotomy defect with methyl methacrylate is an alternative solution.

4.6.7 Pitfalls and Complications

- Injury or thrombosis of the sigmoid sinus
- Injury of the vertebral artery
- CSF fistula
- Caudal cranial nerve injury

References

1. Yasargil MG, Fox JL. The microsurgical approach to intracranial aneurysms. Surg Neurol. 1975;3:7–14.
2. Szelényi A, Langer D, Kothbauer K, De Camargo AB, Flamm ES, Deletis V. Monitoring of muscle motor evoked potentials during cerebral aneurysm surgery: intraoperative changes and postoperative outcome. J Neurosurg. 2006;105:675–81.
3. Schmid-Elsaesser R, Muacevic A, Holtmannspötter M, Uhl E, Steiger HJ. Neuronavigation based on CT angiography for surgery of intracranial aneurysms: primary experience with unruptured aneurysms. Minim Invasive Neurosurg. 2003;46:269–77.
4. Son YJ, Han DH, Kim JE. Image-guided surgery for treatment of unruptured middle cerebral artery aneurysms. Neurosurgery. 2007;61:266–71.
5. Steiger HJ, Schmid-Elsaesser R, Stummer W, Uhl E. Transorbital keyhole approach to anterior communicating artery aneurysms. Neurosurgery. 2001;48: 347–51; discussion 351–2.
6. Beseoglu K, Lodes S, Stummer W, Steiger HJ, Hänggi D. The transorbital keyhole approach: early and long-term outcome analysis of approach-related morbidity and cosmetic results. Technical note. J Neurosurg. 2011;114:852–6.
7. Lehecka M, Dashti R, Hernesniemi J, Niemelä M, Koivisto T, Ronkainen A, et al. Microneurosurgical management of aneurysms at the A2 segment of anterior cerebral artery (proximal pericallosal artery) and its frontobasal branches. Surg Neurol. 2008;70: 232–46.
8. Tsutsumi K, Shiokawa Y, Sakai T, Aoki N, Kubota M, Saito I. Venous infarction following the interhemispheric approach in patients with acute subarachnoid hemorrhage. J Neurosurg. 1991;74:715–9.
9. Nathal E, Gomez-Amador JL. Anatomic and surgical basis of the sphenoid ridge keyhole approach for cerebral aneurysms. Neurosurgery. 2005;56:178–85.
10. Yasargil MG, Reichman MV, Kubik S. Preservation of the frontotemporal branch of the facial nerve using the interfascial temporalis flap for pterional craniotomy. Technical article. J Neurosurg. 1987;67:463–6.
11. Figueiredo EG, Deshmukh P, Nakaji P, Crusius MU, Crawford N, Spetzler RF, et al. The minipterional craniotomy: technical description and anatomic assessment. Neurosurgery. 2007;61:256–64.
12. Kim E, Delashaw Jr JB. Osteoplastic pterional craniotomy revisited. Neurosurgery. 2011;68:125–9.
13. McLaughlin N, Cutler A, Martin NA. Technical nuances of temporal muscle dissection and reconstruction for the pterional keyhole craniotomy. J Neurosurg. 2013;118:309–14.
14. D'Ambrosio AL, Kreiter KT, Bush CA, Sciacca RR, Mayer SA, Solomon RA, et al. Far lateral suboccipital approach for the treatment of proximal posteroinferior cerebellar artery aneurysms: surgical results and long-term outcome. Neurosurgery. 2004;55:39–50; discussion 50–4.
15. Rodríguez-Hernández A, Lawton MT. Anatomical triangles defining surgical routes to posterior inferior cerebellar artery aneurysms. J Neurosurg. 2011;114: 1088–94.

5 Dissection of the Aneurysm and Principles of Clipping

5.1 Approach to the Aneurysm

When operating early after subarachnoid hemorrhage, the anatomy may be much obscured by the cisternal and superficial blood accumulation and by the reactive swelling. It is of utmost importance to ensure sufficient brain relaxation prior to opening the dura. The ventricular or spinal CSF drain should be opened following craniotomy and 50–100 mL of CSF should be drained. It is important not to open the dura while it is still under tension, because doing so could result in brain prolapse and premature rerupture of the aneurysm. At this point, it is also important to check arterial pressure and communicate with the anesthesiologist. We recommend keeping the arterial pressure at a level corresponding to the preoperative value minus the preoperatively measured intracranial pressure (ICP). If preoperative ICP levels are not available, 10 mmHg is used as an average estimate, and arterial pressure during surgery should therefore be maintained at 10 mmHg lower than the preoperative value. This directive keeps the cerebral perfusion pressure steady, thus both avoiding ischemia and controlling the risk of premature rerupture of the aneurysm.

5.2 Opening the Cisterns

Once the dura has been opened, the aim is to gain proximal control and free the neck of the aneurysm with as little dissection as possible. Any dissection in the vicinity of the aneurysm carries the risk of rupture. The only location where the fragile aneurysm dome is not encountered with certainty is the parent artery. Therefore, the parent artery should be identified, and dissection to the aneurysm neck should strictly adhere to this vessel. The parent artery is our friend.

5.3 Gaining Proximal Control

The method of gaining proximal control depends essentially on the specific aneurysm location. It is generally not necessary to dissect the entire parent artery beginning with its origin from the internal carotid artery. In the case of an anterior communicating artery aneurysm, it is sufficient to look for the A1 in its middle segment, at the level where it crosses the optic nerve. In the case of a middle cerebral artery aneurysm (particularly when using the smaller sylvian approach),

H.-J. Steiger et al., *Microsurgical Brain Aneurysms: Illustrated Concepts and Cases*,
DOI 10.1007/978-3-662-45679-8_5, © Springer-Verlag Berlin Heidelberg 2015

the M2 segments are usually identified first in the depth of the sylvian fissure, and these are followed backward to the bifurcation in order to secure inflow from M1 and the aneurysm neck.

Gaining proximal control always provides only relative safety. Complete control of aneurysm inflow, which is necessary to deal with complex aneurysms, can be achieved only by controlling all afferent and efferent arteries. In the case of anterior communicating artery aneurysms, for example, both A1 and A2 segments must be controlled—keeping in mind that sometimes unexpected arteries can be present, such as a third A2 segment.

For noncomplex aneurysms, gaining proximal control is less important than achieving complete understanding of the anatomy of the perianeurysmal vascular complex. Therefore, no efforts should be made to control a contralateral nondominant A1 hiding behind a downward-projecting aneurysm at the anterior communicating artery, for example.

5.4 Dissecting the Neck of the Aneurysm

Having gained access to the parent artery, the neck of the aneurysm is approached along this artery. At this point, the importance of a clear mental image of the expected configuration of the neck in relation to the parent and branching arteries cannot be overemphasized. It is therefore important to study the preoperative 3D reconstructions of the angiography exactly, also from the direction of approach. Nonetheless, details may not be evident from the angiography, so knowledge of the common variations is important. After the widening of the parent artery suggesting that the aneurysmal neck has been defined (Fig. 5.1), both sides of the neck must be separated from the arterial branches sufficiently to allow the smooth passage later of the clip blades (in general, at least 3 mm). The dome of the aneurysm is left untouched at this stage. Separation of the neck from the arteries needs to be complete so that the dissector can be passed through.

Because the back side of the neck is not visible, a common error is to assume that it looks the same as the visible front side, but this may not be the case. The neck may be directed backward from the line of sight, thus bulging on the back side. The other variant, that the aneurysm is projecting somewhat toward the surgeon, is usually more easily realized.

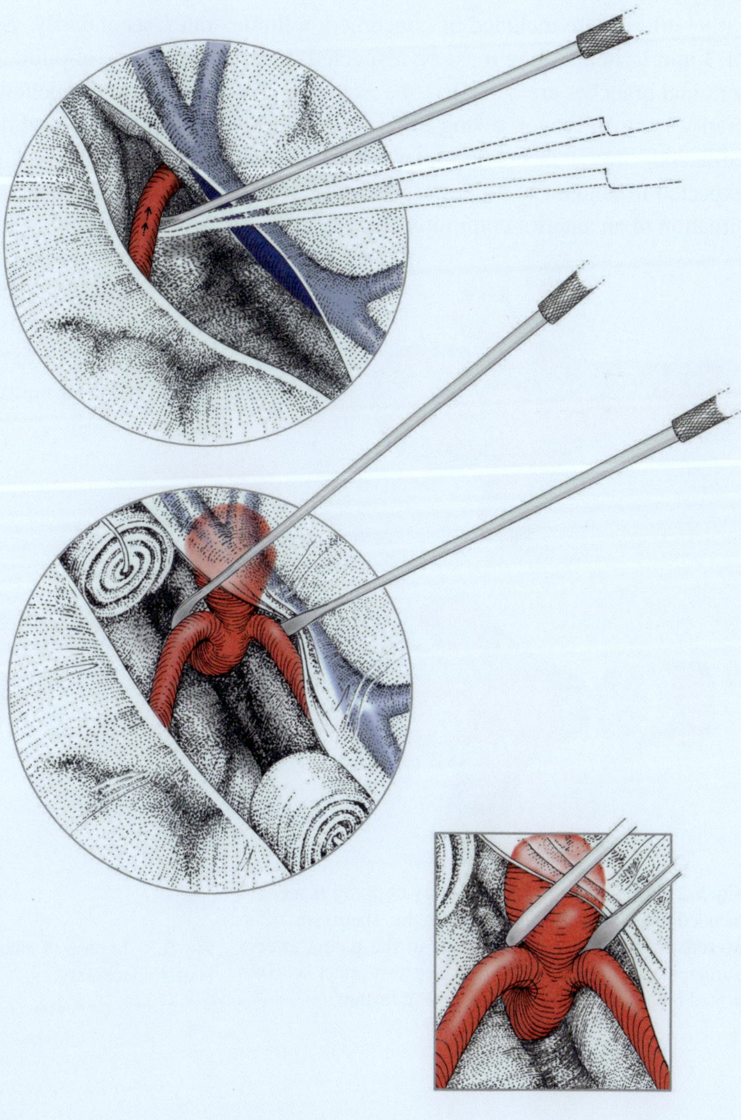

Fig. 5.1 Following identification of the proximal parent artery or a distal branch, this artery is followed to the aneurysm-bearing bifurcation and the aneurysm neck. The neck is subsequently freed on both sides, while leaving the aneurysm dome untouched

5.5 Temporary Clipping, Pharmacological Neuroprotection, and Induced Hypotension

Temporary clipping has proven to be a very useful adjunct for aneurysm clipping [1]. We recommend the general use of proximal temporary clipping whenever the neck of the aneurysm is wider than the parent artery (Fig. 5.2). We do not recommend the use of temporary clipping during dissection as it usually takes considerable time and its benefit is questionable, in our opinion.

Some precautions and caveats need to be mentioned with regard to temporary clipping. The limits of ischemic tolerance in the particular territory need to be kept in mind. Whenever perforating arteries are included or concerned, a limit of 3 min ischemic time must be respected. If no terminal branches are occluded, the ischemic tolerance is much longer, owing to leptomeningeal collateral flow. Ischemic tolerance can be expected to amount to at least 15–20 min in the situation of an anterior communicating or middle cerebral artery aneurysm, as long as the aneurysm does not bleed, which would lead to steal of the leptomeningeal collateral flow. If aneurysm rupture occurs, retrograde drainage of the leptomeningeal collateral flow needs to be blocked by completely trapping the aneurysm, thus also clamping the efferent arteries (Fig. 5.3).

Although it is difficult to prove in a stringent manner, there is little doubt that neuroprotective drugs can prolong ischemic tolerance. The use of barbiturates or similar drugs is not justified in the case of a simple aneurysm for which a temporary clipping time of only a few minutes is expected. In these situations, we recommend starting without pharmacological protection. If the period of temporary clipping turns out to last longer than expected, we start the administration of barbiturates secondarily. Specifically, after 10 min of temporary clipping, we administer a bolus of 500 mg of thiopental, and after that 100 mg every 2 min, until a total dose of 2 g has been given. If neurophysiological monitoring is available, we increase the dose until burst suppression is achieved and maintain this state until blood flow has been restored. This approach is admittedly open to question, because according to common logic the drug should be given prior to temporary clipping in order to reach the target territory. The major effect of neurodepressive neuroprotection,

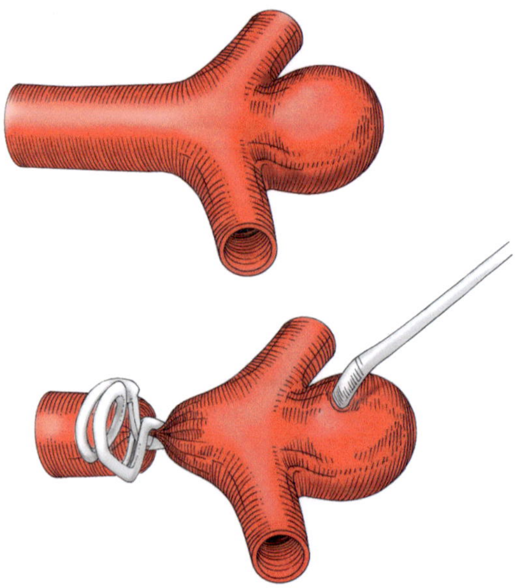

Fig. 5.2 Primary proximal temporary clipping is recommended whenever the diameter of the aneurysm neck exceeds the physiological diameter of the parent artery. Sufficient decompression of the aneurysm must be confirmed by palpation prior to proceeding further

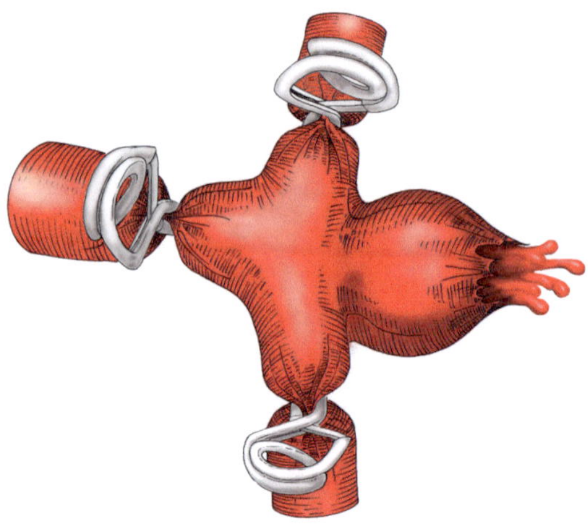

Fig. 5.3 In case of aneurysm rupture, complete trapping is often necessary

however, may well lie in the reduction of blood flow in the neighboring territories, thus increasing leptomeningeal collateral flow.

If long temporary occlusion times are expected (i.e., with complex aneurysms), it is certainly reasonable to induce pharmacological neuroprotection prior to temporary clipping.

In some situations, the use of temporary induced hypotension is useful. For example, in case of a carotid ophthalmic artery aneurysm, the possibilities of depressurizing the aneurysm by proximal control are insufficient, and a short period of controlled hypotension is necessary to prevent aneurysm rupture during clip application [2].

5.6 Pilot Clipping

Following sufficient dissection of the aneurysm neck, a clip that is expected to fit best is selected from the supply. It is important to measure the diameter of the neck on the angiogram. The necessary clip length will correspond to the diameter multiplied by $\pi/2$. If this measurement is smaller than the size that appears necessary from intraoperative perception, the conclusion must be that the structure perceived intraoperatively as the aneurysm neck does not correspond to only the neck but may also include a brain artery.

The philosophy of clipping has changed considerably over the past decades. Most companies provide a wide range of different configurations in order to optimally model the vascular contour. This idea is certainly compelling, but complex configurations have disadvantages. These clips can be applied only in one specific way and in one defined final position. They cannot be advanced a bit more or less, as a straight clip can, for example, nor can complex clips be rotated. In short, complex configurations limit the degrees of freedom during application (Fig. 5.4). Moreover, if the shape of the neck turns out to differ somewhat from the expectation, the complex clip must be removed completely and replaced by a better-fitting configuration. Finally, complex configurations are bulkier than straight or slightly curved clips and therefore are often awkward to manage in small surgical access channels. For these reasons, we prefer to use simple straight or slightly curved clip shapes and then add additional small clips to exclude residual dog ears.

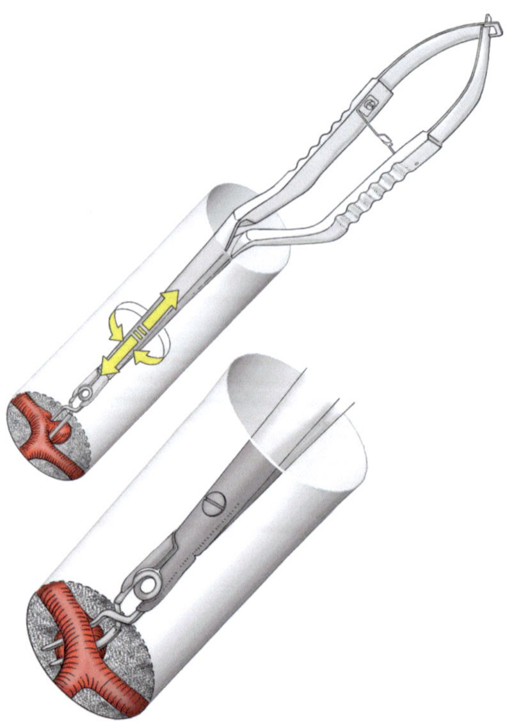

Fig. 5.4 Using straight or slightly curved clips permits at least two degrees of freedom, whereas complex aneurysm clips can be applied in just one way. Furthermore, complex configurations require more maneuvering space and are therefore often impractical in narrow surgical fields

Applying the pilot clip needs to be done carefully and slowly. If the clip blades do not slide smoothly across the neck, either prior dissection has been insufficient or the anatomical concept is wrong—that is, the clip is blocked by part of the aneurysm or the parent artery or a branch. If this happens, the clip must be removed and the situation clarified.

After passing the blades completely across the neck, the clip is slowly released. Application of the pilot clip is the time when intraoperative aneurysm rupture most commonly occurs [3]. Releasing the clip slowly makes it possible to realize if the aneurysm is tacked somewhere. Slow release of the clip also prevents a large tear of the fundus or, even worse, at the base of the neck.

The behavior of the clip after release is important and should be recorded. If the clip twists out of the direction of application, this is a telltale sign that something is between the clip blades on the back side that does not belong there (usually an arterial branch).

Bleeding from the aneurysm at any stage requires control. With smaller aneurysms, control is achieved by putting a cotton patty on the leak and applying gentle compression. With larger leaks or larger aneurysms, the situation calls for complete trapping of the aneurysm with temporary clipping of all afferent and efferent arteries.

5.7 Final Solutions

If the initial clip has been managed uneventfully across the neck and released, it is not yet time to step back and relax. Now that the clip has opened the view to the back side, each blade must be carefully inspected to see that it crosses the neck completely and does not include adjacent perforators (Fig. 5.5). The clip should be freely movable together with the aneurysm. Otherwise the clip has caught something it should not, possibly an arterial branch. If incomplete clipping of the neck or trapping of a cerebral artery has been noticed, the solution is to apply a second, parallel clip a bit higher on the dome and then to correct the initial clip or replace it with one of a different configuration (more curved).

At the end, the final clip should completely cross the neck and not trap any perforators. Small dog-ears at the base should be eliminated by additional small clips.

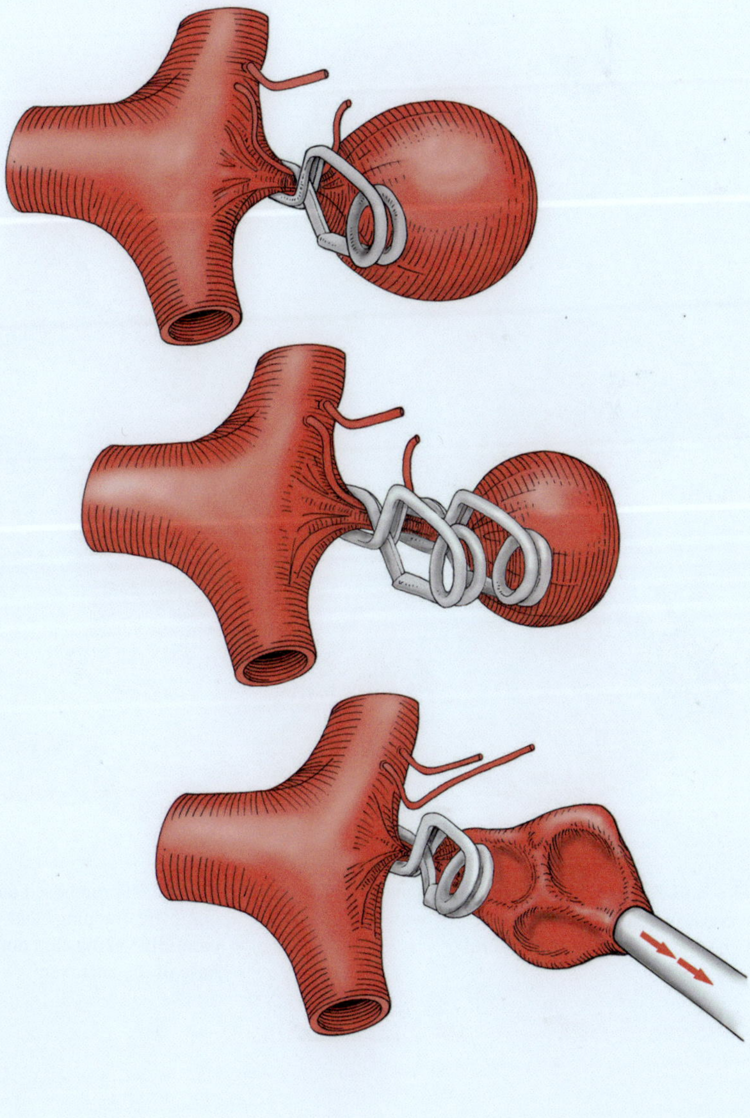

Fig. 5.5 Provisional application of a pilot clip. When the pilot clip has been released, it must be inspected to look for incomplete crossing of the neck or trapped perforators. Correction is accomplished by application of a second, parallel clip and subsequent replacement of the initial clip

5.8 Complex Solutions

Large and complex aneurysms require complex solutions using multiple clips [4–6]. For a broad-necked aneurysm, the simplest variant is tandem clipping, initially using a fenestrated clip for the distal portion of the neck and then a straight clip for the proximal part (Fig. 5.6). This solution was more important when closing forces of clips were more limited and were insufficient for large aneurysms. Today, only giant aneurysms still challenge the closing forces of the available clips and require a tandem technique or the application of several parallel clips.

Partially thrombosed aneurysms need to be opened and the thrombus must be carefully removed in an endarterectomy-like fashion (Fig. 5.7). Fusiform and dissecting aneurysms need to be wrapped or trapped (Fig. 5.8). If trapping involves an insufficiently collateralized vascular segment, flow replacement by bypass surgery becomes necessary. However, the need for bypass surgery must be settled prior to surgery, as ad hoc indications and ad hoc bypass procedures after unplanned occlusion of an important artery are prone to failure and may not save the situation.

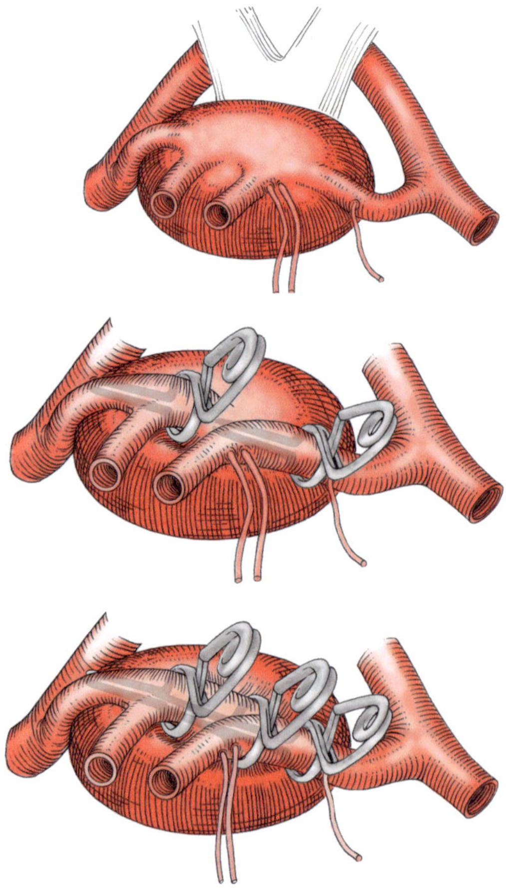

Fig. 5.6 Broad-based and complex aneurysms require reconstruction of the parent vessel with multiple clips. Fenestrated clips are often useful

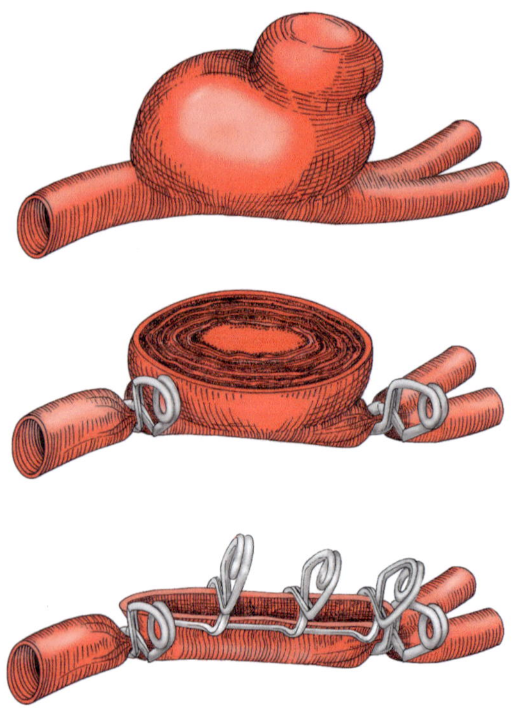

Fig. 5.7 Thrombosed aneurysms need to be opened after complete trapping, and the thrombus must be removed carefully, taking care not to perforate the outer wall at the base of the aneurysm

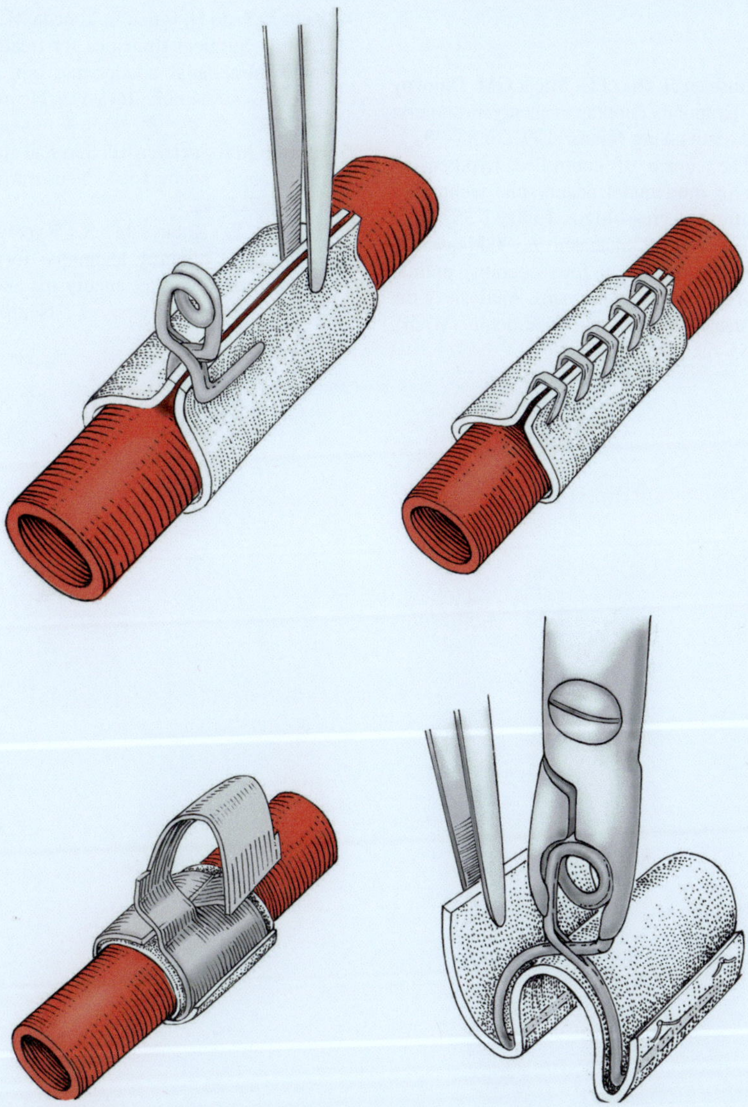

Fig. 5.8 Fusiform and dissecting aneurysms can be secured by wrapping with Teflon or Dacron sheets or with the help of encircling clips

References

1. Charbel FT, Ausman JI, Diaz FG, Malik GM, Dujovny M, Sanders J. Temporary clipping in aneurysm surgery: technique and results. Surg Neurol. 1991;36:83–90.
2. Lam AM. The choice of controlled hypotension during repair of intracranial aneurysms: techniques and complications. Agressologie. 1990;31:357–9.
3. Houkin K, Kuroda S, Takahashi A, Takikawa S, Ishikawa T, Yoshimoto T, et al. Intra-operative premature rupture of the cerebral aneurysms. Analysis of the causes and management. Acta Neurochir (Wien). 1999;141:1255–63.
4. Kato Y, Sano H, Imizu S, Yoneda M, Viral M, Nagata J, et al. Surgical strategies for treatment of giant or large intracranial aneurysms: our experience with 139 cases. Minim Invasive Neurosurg. 2003;46: 339–43.
5. Lawton MT, Spetzler RF. Surgical strategies for giant intracranial aneurysms. Neurosurg Clin N Am. 1998;9:725–42.
6. Tanaka Y, Kobayashi S, Kyoshima K, Sugita K. Multiple clipping technique for large and giant internal carotid artery aneurysms and complications: angiographic analysis. J Neurosurg. 1994;80: 635–42.

6 Aneurysms of the Anterior Cerebral Artery

6.1 Anterior Communicating Artery Aneurysms

6.1.1 General Considerations

As described earlier in this book, anterior communicating artery aneurysms are best classified on hemodynamic grounds into four types according to the projection of the dome. The projection of the dome determines to a large degree specific problems of the approach and the manner of clip application:

- Type 1 aneurysms project downward to the optic chiasm and often adhere to this structure. This adherence is important because elevating the orbital cortex with a brain retractor during the approach may lead to traction on the aneurysm dome and to premature intraoperative rerupture.
- Type 2 aneurysms project essentially forward as an elongation of the dominant A1 segment. Although they do not adhere to the chiasm, they lie within the interhemispheric fissure, so formal splitting of the fissure between the gyri recti is therefore hazardous with these aneurysms.
- The dome of type 3 aneurysms lies approximately within the plane of the A2 segments. Although the initial approach is less problematic than with the type 1 and 2 projections, type 3 aneurysms require more upward dissection and retraction, owing to the higher position of the aneurysm neck. Furthermore, type 3 aneurysms are close to the perforators originating from distal A1 and proximal A2 segments.
- Type 4 aneurysms lie above the plane of the A1 segments and behind the plane of the A2s. These aneurysms require access to the neck above the A1s, which is between perforators. Type 4 aneurysms are also close to the hypothalamus, and this structure is hurt by aneurysmal hemorrhage and surgical manipulations more easily than with the other projections. Therefore, type 4 projections are associated with a less favorable functional outcome than the other projections.

Of course, the other important variable that determines the complexity of surgical obliteration and outcome is aneurysm size. It is unclear whether the effect of size on surgical problems and outcome is different than for other anterior circulation sites, but it appears likely that this is indeed the case. That is, giant anterior communicating artery aneurysms have a worse outcome than giant middle cerebral artery aneurysms.

6.1.2 Dissection of Anterior Communicating Artery Aneurysms and Clipping

The orbitocranial approach is favored for all anterior communicating artery aneurysms, as outlined earlier. Prior to opening the dura, sufficient brain relaxation is achieved by drainage of

H.-J. Steiger et al., *Microsurgical Brain Aneurysms: Illustrated Concepts and Cases*,
DOI 10.1007/978-3-662-45679-8_6, © Springer-Verlag Berlin Heidelberg 2015

50–100 mL of CSF, in case of subarachnoid hemorrhage (SAH) by a lumbar or ventricular drain and by mannitol if necessary (1–2 g/kg body weight). Following gentle elevation of the orbital cortex and opening the central aspect of the sylvian fissure, further steps depend on the aneurysm projection. In any case, the next waypoint is the optic nerve. The small retractor blade that is usually necessary for this approach must be pointing to the ipsilateral optic nerve. This strategy prevents severing the aneurysm with the retractor blade because the anterior communicating artery and the aneurysms almost always lie completely in front of the optic nerve. Nonetheless, care is mandatory even when the retractor blade is not put in front of the chiasm, particularly with a type 1 projection, where the dome of the aneurysm often adheres to the anterior aspect of the chiasm.

Following insertion of the blade, the prechiasmatic cistern is opened medial to the now-opened sylvian fissure. Finally, the cistern must be opened all the way medially to the interhemispheric fissure to allow mobilization of the straight gyrus and access to the A1 segment. At this stage, the surgeon must decide how to proceed. Medial opening of the prechiasmatic cistern and splitting the proximal interhemispheric fissure can be done safely with aneurysm projections type 3 and 4. The interhemispheric arachnoid adhesions can be separated by using bipolar forceps with a spreading motion, as usually done to split the sylvian fissure [1]. Care is required with ventral (type 1) and anterior (type 2) projections. A straight anterior projection of the aneurysm dome renders formal splitting of the interhemispheric fissure dangerous. In these situations, it may be more appropriate to perform a small resection of the gyrus rectus medial to the olfactory tract.

These steps allow further mobilization of the orbital cortex. The posterior aspect of the gyrus rectus is now separated from the chiasm. The A1 segment of the anterior cerebral artery must be identified at this stage. The artery should be looked for at the point where it crosses the optic nerve (Fig. 6.1). It is not necessary to follow the artery to its origin from the internal carotid artery. When the artery has been identified, the back side must be dissected locally in order to apply a temporary clip, in case clipping should become urgently necessary. Attention must also be paid to the retrograde Heubner's artery, which originates on the ventrolateral aspect of the A2 origin and then retrogradely parallels the A1 segment along its dorsal circumference.

The exposure can now be stabilized prior to further dissection. To distribute the pressure on the orbital cortex, it is helpful to insert a rolled cottonoid in front of the spatula between the orbital roof and the orbital cortex. During this maneuver, attention must be paid to the olfactory bulb.

A few words shall be spent regarding opening of the lamina terminalis, which now comes into the surgical field. If there is functioning ventricular or spinal CSF drainage, opening the lamina terminalis does not add much with regard to brain relaxation. If operative access has been achieved without external CSF drainage, opening the lamina terminalis certainly helps to relax the brain. Other benefits have been postulated, such as minimizing postoperative hydrocephalus or vasospasm, but convincing proof has not been provided.

The A1 is now followed anteriorly to the anterior communicating artery. With high-running A1s, a certain problem often occurs at this stage. It may become necessary to further split the interhemispheric fissure or to perform some medial resection of the straight gyrus. A limited resection is not known to have any negative consequences. Applying undue retraction with the retractor blade, on the other hand, must be avoided not only because of brain damage but also because it is usually a futile effort to achieve sufficient exposure in cases of insufficient dissection.

Following identification and dissection of the A1-A2 transition, the further steps depend essentially on the type of projection. If it is easily possible, the surgeon should now attempt to achieve complete control of afferent blood flow—that is, to identify the contralateral A1 and prepare it for temporary clipping. In case of type 1 projection, however, this is usually not feasible and should be omitted. With the other projections, however, the contralateral (usually hypoplastic) A1 should be controlled at this stage. The direction of the contralateral A1 is usually straight up toward the surgeon. The artery should be dissected segmentally in order to apply a temporary clip. The origin of the contralateral A2 is commonly hidden behind the aneurysm; it is therefore difficult to identify at this stage, and no effort should be made to do so. Identification of the contralateral A2 becomes easier after dissection of the aneurysm neck. Sometimes, however, the contralateral A2 can be visualized only after applying a clip on the aneurysm neck. During dissection of the A2 segments, the origin of Heubner's artery needs special attention and must be spared.

It is worthwhile to quickly review the specific pathoanatomy with regard to the A2 segments. Physiological elongation of the A1 segments during aging leads normally to a rotation of the anterior communicating artery so that the origin of A2 on the side of the larger A1 is displaced posteriorly. In our experience, this configuration is found in approximately 80 % of all patients with an anterior communicating artery aneurysm. In the remaining 20 %, however, the origin of the A2 is displaced anteriorly on the side of the dominant A1. As nicely pointed out by Suzuki and colleagues [2], this configuration poses an additional surgical difficulty as the contralateral A2 is hiding behind the ipsilateral one. This so-called closed configuration results also in a distinctly worse functional outcome than with the so-called open A2 configuration, in which the contralateral A2 can be easily identified in front of the ipsilateral A2.

Now that proximal control has been gained, the further steps are dissection of the aneurysm neck and clip application, as outlined earlier. With inferiorly projecting aneurysms (type 1), both sides of the neck are dissected in front beneath the anterior communicating artery (Fig. 6.2). With anterior projecting aneurysms (type 2), necessary neck dissection may be limited to the space in front of the anterior communicating artery (Fig. 6.3), but sometimes with a wide neck, the origins of the A2s stick to the neck and must be freed. As mentioned, identification and separation of the contralateral A2 may not be easy at this stage, and the situation may need clarification after applying a pilot clip on the aneurysm neck. Corresponding to the dissection, both clip branches are then passed beneath or in front of the anterior communicating artery, essentially parallel to the plane of the anterior communicating artery. Straight aneurysm clips usually fit well for type 1 and type 2 projections (Fig. 6.4). As mentioned before, we recommend temporary clipping of the ipsilateral A1 whenever the aneurysm neck is wider than the A1 diameter.

Following application of the pilot clip, the situs is now closely inspected. Both branches are checked to see that the aneurysm neck is completely obliterated and a cerebral artery has not been trapped. Now the contralateral A2 origin must be identified. If the clip has grasped the contralateral A2, a second parallel clip should be applied a bit higher on the aneurysm neck. The first clip can then be corrected, possibly after additional dissection of the A2 origin and separation from the neck. Anatomic variations of the A2 segments must be kept in mind at this stage. The most common error is to ignore the situation in which there are three A2 segments.

At the end, appropriate flow in all vascular segments is confirmed by indocyanine green (ICG) videoangiography, micro-Doppler, or both.

Aneurysms lying between the A2 segments (type 3) pose other challenges for dissection and clipping. Here dissection of the aneurysm neck involves separation of the A2 origins from the neck (Fig. 6.5). This is best achieved with a small dissector or blunt microhook. In the open A2 configuration, as outlined above, both sides can be seen (Fig. 6.6). In contrast, with the closed configuration, the contralateral A2 passes behind the aneurysm, and separation prior to clipping is challenging or even impossible without applying a pilot clip on the aneurysm. Once satisfactory separation has been achieved, a pilot clip corresponding to the expected neck size (diameter on angiogram $\times \pi/2$) is carefully applied. With the open A2 configuration, the clip direction is approximately perpendicular to the plane of the A2s. With the closed configuration, the clip direction will be somewhat oblique with regard to the A2 plane. For a right-sided approach, it is usually best to apply the clip with the left hand, and vice versa.

The further steps are essentially identical to those described for types 1 and 2. If the location of A2 is unclear prior to application of the clip, it needs to be localized now. With the closed A2 configuration, it may happen that the contralateral A2 gets included between the clip blades. This is corrected by applying a second parallel clip a bit higher on the aneurysm and subsequently replacing the first clip.

A particular problem with the type 3 projection is that the posterior aspect of the aneurysm neck is commonly underestimated. It often bulges considerably on the back side, more than anticipated from the front aspect. If not accounted for, an aneurysm residue will remain at the posterior aspect. Using a downward curved clip instead of a straight one solves this problem (Fig. 6.7).

Type 4 aneurysms of the anterior communicating artery lie behind the A2s and above the A1s (Fig. 6.8). They require extensive mobilization of the straight gyrus and usually removal of some tissue. Access and dissection of the aneurysm neck must be done above the anterior communicating artery. Particular attention must be paid to the perforators and to Heubner's artery. Following complete dissection of both sides of the neck, clipping and further evaluation are essentially the same as with types 1 and 2, with the difference, of course, that the clip is passed on the back side of the anterior communicating artery (Fig. 6.9).

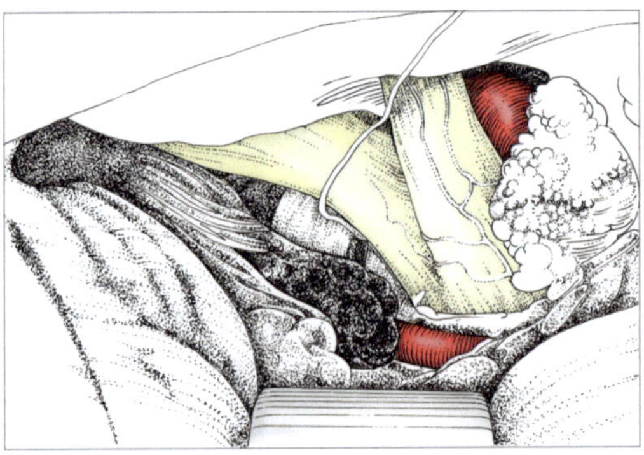

Fig. 6.1 Ventrally projecting anterior communicating aneurysm (type 1) approached from the right. Identifying A1 at the level of the optic nerve

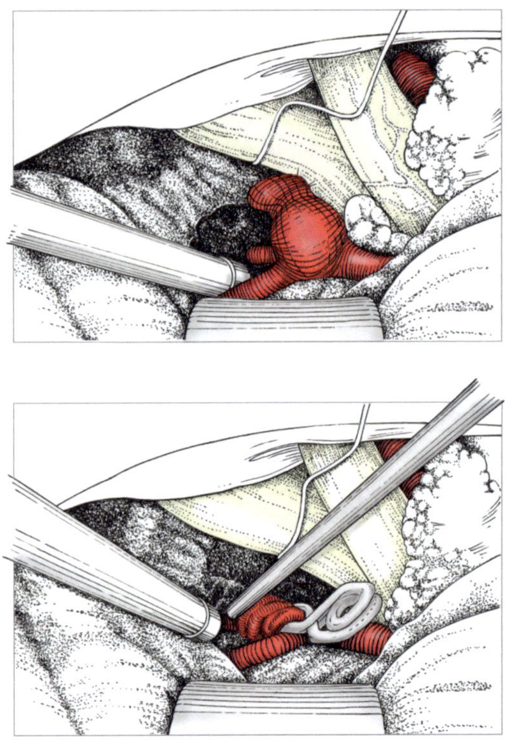

Fig. 6.2 Dissecting the aneurysm and identifying both A2 segments. The white material on the right of the chiasm is a gelatin pledget. Clipping and verification of adequate flow in both A2s by means of the micro-Doppler probe

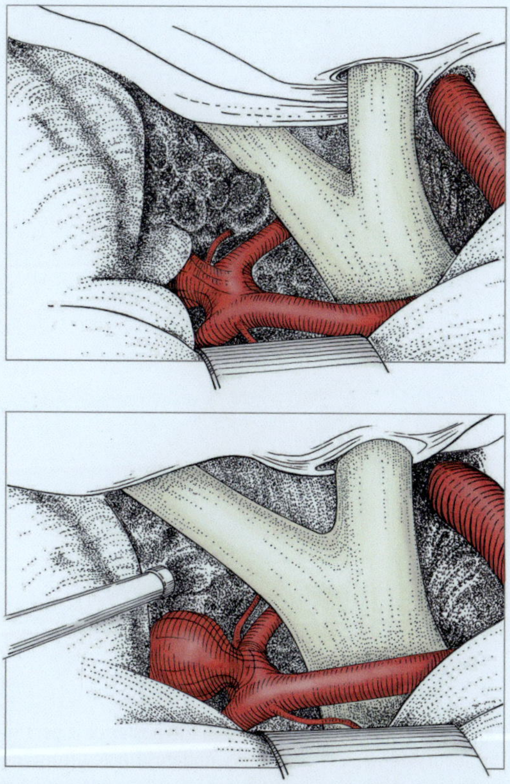

Fig. 6.3 Anteriorly projecting anterior communicating aneurysm (type 2) approached from the right. Surgical field following careful removal of cisternal clot

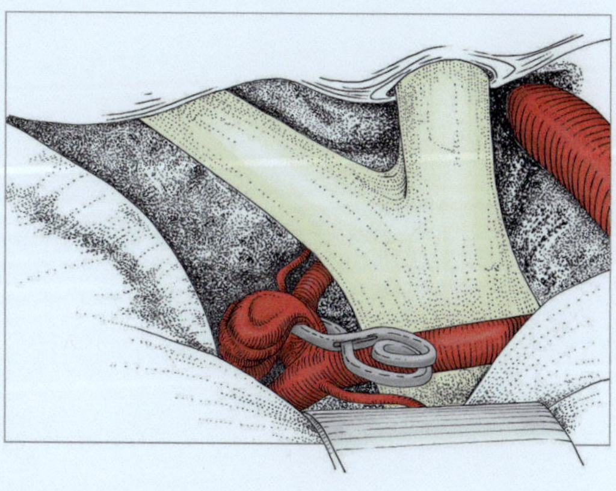

Fig. 6.4 Clipping with a straight clip parallel to the anterior communicating artery

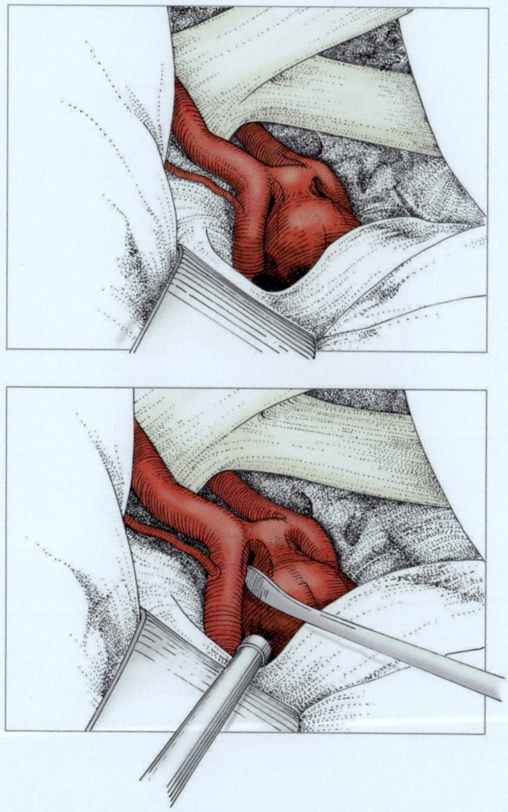

Fig. 6.5 Anterior communicating artery aneurysm (type 3) lying between the A2 segments, approached from the left. Dissecting the neck and separation from the adjacent A2 origins

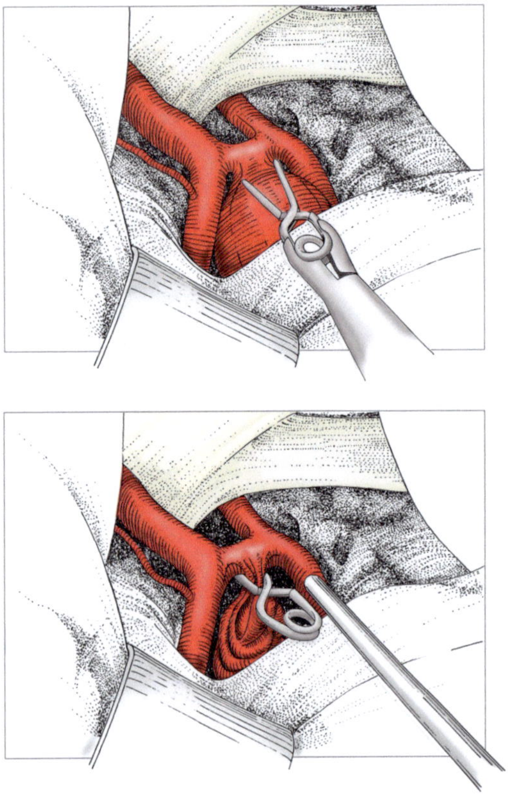

Fig. 6.6 Clip application. Verifying appropriate flow in the A2 segments with a micro-Doppler probe

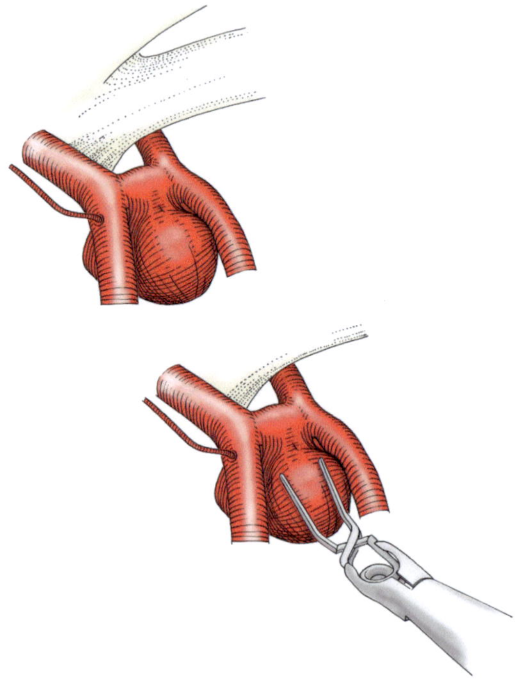

Fig. 6.7 With a type 3 projection, the posterior aspect of the aneurysm neck is commonly underestimated from the front view. Use of a curved clip may be necessary for complete clipping

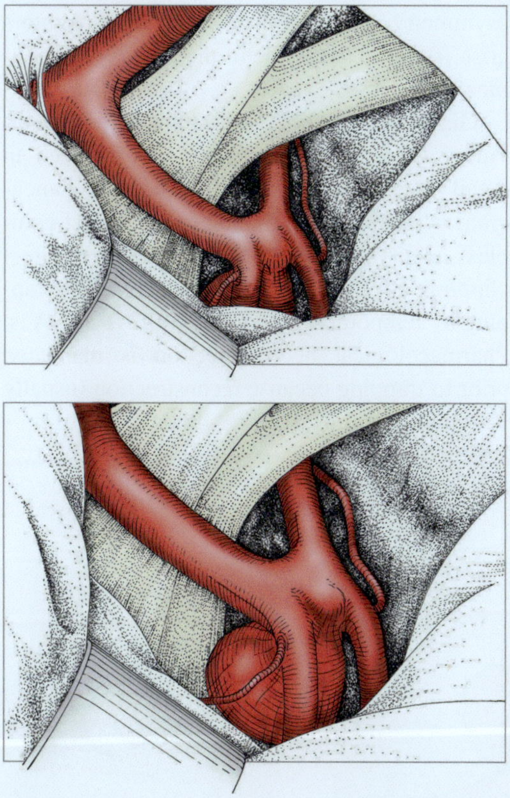

Fig. 6.8 Anterior communicating artery aneurysm (type 4) lying behind the A2 segments, approached from the left. The aneurysm dome lies behind the A2 segments and requires dissection above the anterior communicating artery

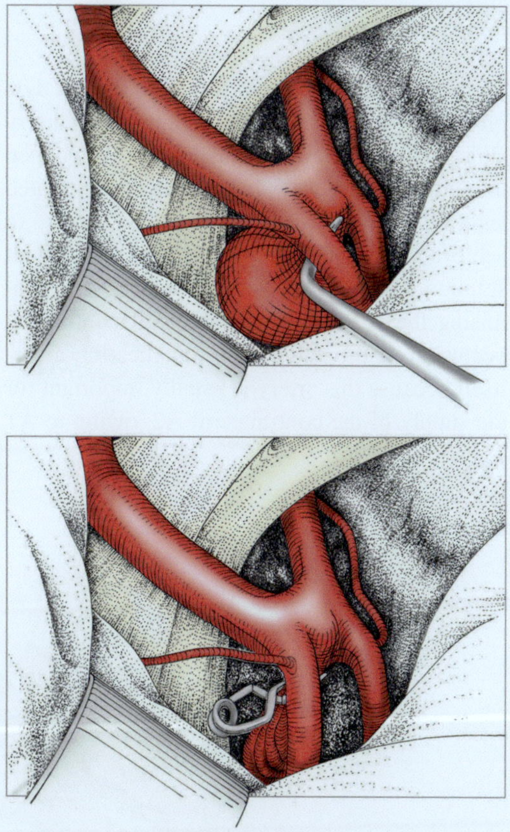

Fig. 6.9 Dissection of the neck from behind the A1-A2 transition. The clip is also applied behind the A1-A2 transition

6.1.3 Special Cases

Sometimes several bulges originate from a dysplastically dilated anterior communicating artery (Fig. 6.10). The different bulges must be clipped individually with partial inclusion of the dilated anterior communicating artery in order to achieve a more physiologic diameter. A perfect solution is not always possible without compromising the A2 origins. We do not recommend occlusion of the anterior communicating artery itself because this artery is usually important for the supply of the contralateral A2, owing to A1 asymmetry, and also because some perforators arise from the back side of the anterior communicating artery.

Giant and complex aneurysms require individual strategies that cannot be formalized in detail [3–5]. It must be decided whether the aneurysm is amenable to direct clipping. Most complex aneurysms can be addressed by direct clipping, but the process requires complete trapping by temporary clipping of both A1 and A2s. Pharmacological neuroprotection is mandated prior to trapping because reconstruction (usually with multiple clips) requires time.

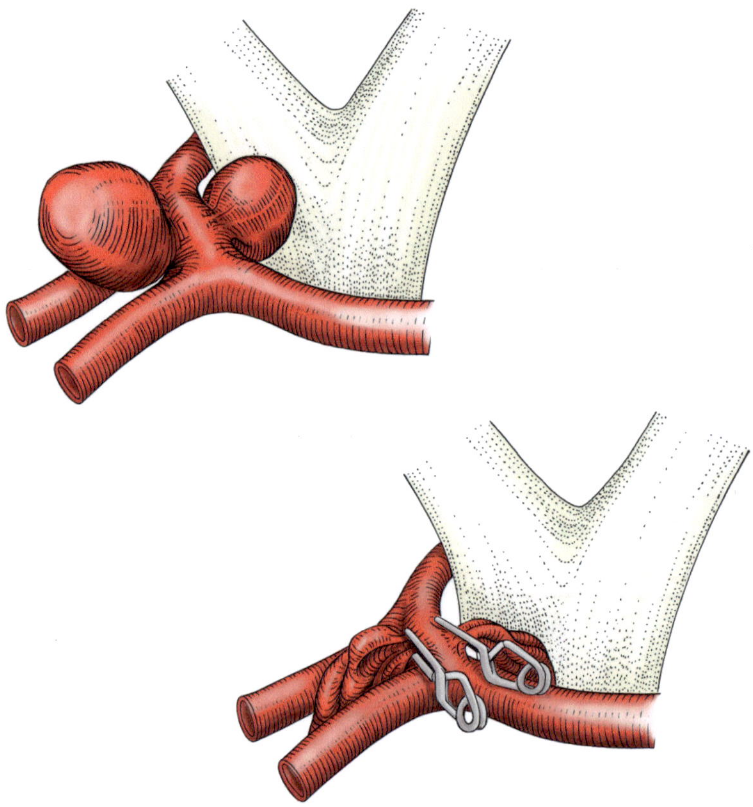

Fig. 6.10 Multiple aneurysms may arise from a dysplastic anterior communicating artery. The bulges are clipped individually

6.2 A2–Pericallosal Artery Aneurysms

6.2.1 General Considerations

Distal anterior cerebral artery aneurysms originate most often at the origin of the pericallosal artery. They are relatively rare, with proportions reported from 1 to 3 % of intracranial aneurysms. Although not as well known as the anterior communicating artery aneurysm, asymmetry of the afferent arteries plays a pathophysiological role. Huber et al. [6] and Perlmutter and Rhoton [7] pointed out that the situation of an unpaired A2 segment (azygos A2) particularly is associated with a high risk of developing an aneurysm at the origin of the pericallosal artery.

Pericallosal artery aneurysms are considered primary candidates for a microsurgical approach because of their relatively peripheral location, although this concept is increasingly challenged by advanced endovascular techniques [8]. With regard to the surgical approach, there are no alternatives to the interhemispheric route. This approach, however, is all but trivial [9, 10]. Results of surgical treatment of pericallosal artery aneurysms were worse than with other locations. The early series published by Thomas and Paterson [11] reported roughly 25 % mortality and 25 % morbidity for a patient group managed prior to the advent of early surgery after SAH. The reasons must be retrospectively seen in the lack of image guidance at that time (resulting in larger and more traumatic approaches), the lack of CSF drainage resulting in retraction injury, venous injury associated with larger approaches, and finally the high risk of vasospastic complications at this location.

These dangers and complications define the focus of today's minimally invasive surgical procedures. The variability of the origin of the pericallosal artery mandates the use of image-guided navigation. A lumbar CSF drain is mandatory for unruptured aneurysms, because the approach does not offer early access to CSF spaces that could be drained in order to achieve sufficient brain relaxation.

The details of the approach have been described in the first part of this book, but we shall repeat here a few thoughts with regard to the choice of the side of the craniotomy. Because the falx cerebri ends approximately 2 cm above the corpus callosum, both pericallosal arteries can be reached from either side. The projection of the typical pericallosal artery aneurysm is oriented close to the sagittal plane, but some aneurysms project more toward the cingulate gyrus (often associated with intracerebral hemorrhage), and some aneurysms point more to the midline. We plan the approach based on the angiogram and the 3-D reconstruction in order to achieve direct access to the base without the need to maneuver around the dome. In case of intracerebral hematoma, we recommend choosing the side of the hematoma for the approach. This concept is arguable, however, because the principally intraparenchymal hematoma arising from a pericallosal artery aneurysm can also be evacuated from the contralateral side.

6.2.2 Dissection of Pericallosal Artery Aneurysms and Clipping

After identification of the distal pericallosal artery, the dissection advances proximally on the artery to the neck of the aneurysm and the callosomarginal artery (Fig. 6.11). The neck of an aneurysm on the distal side usually can be easily separated from the distal pericallosal artery. On the other hand, the neck along the origin of the pericallosal artery is often quite broad. Here care is required in separating the pericallosal artery from the proximal neck.

Following appropriate dissection of the neck, the aneurysm is clipped, using a clip configuration chosen on the basis of the preoperative imaging and the intraoperative perspective. It is often helpful to use an upward-curved clip or an angled clip, owing to the orientation of the neck (Fig. 6.12). Following application of the pilot clip, the situs is carefully inspected along the blades to ascertain complete obliteration and preservation of the parent arteries. As mentioned, these aneurysms are often broad based, and perfect elimination without compromising the callosomarginal artery may not be possible. If micro-Doppler and/or ICG angiography show that the flow in the pericallosal artery is compromised, a parallel clip should be applied a bit higher on the dome. The resulting dog-ear toward the distal pericallosal artery after removal of the first clip may be eliminated by an additional small clip.

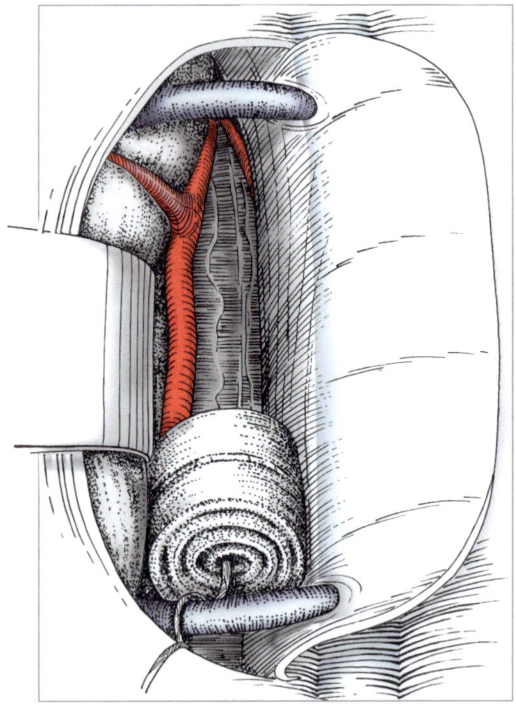

Fig. 6.11 The initial interhemispheric view following left-sided approach to a right pericallosal artery aneurysm, with identification of the left and right supracallosal segments of the pericallosal arteries

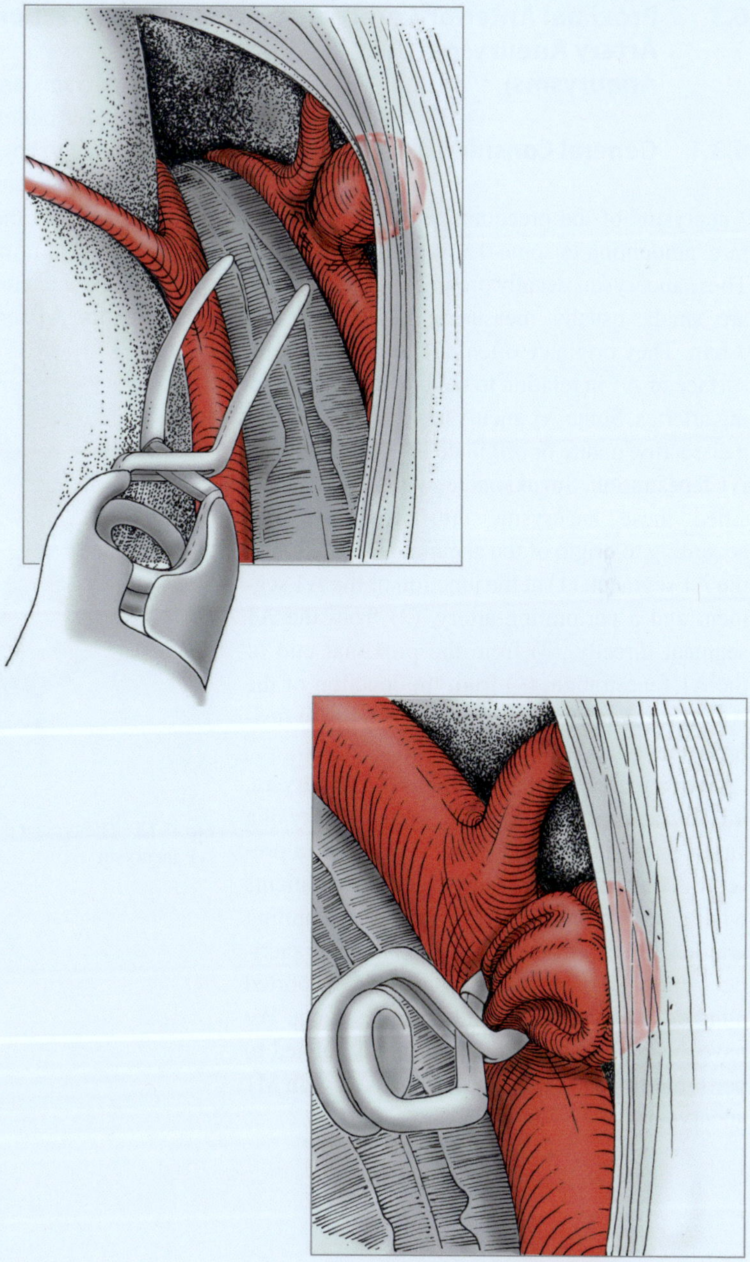

Fig. 6.12 Clipping with a curved clip following identification and dissection of the neck. Inspection to ensure complete clipping and patency of the pericallosal artery

6.2.3 Special Cases

As Huber and colleagues [6] pointed out, asymmetry of the A2 segments (and particularly the situation of an unpaired A2 segment) plays a role in the formation of aneurysms at the origin of the pericallosal artery. The unpaired pericallosal artery (so-called azygos A2) supplies bilateral cortical areas. From the viewpoint of surgical approach and microsurgical technique, the condition has little impact except for the larger territory at risk.

6.3 Proximal Anterior Cerebral Artery Aneurysms (A1 Aneurysms)

6.3.1 General Considerations

Aneurysms of the precommunicating artery are rare, amounting to some 0.5 % of all aneurysms. These aneurysms usually present with SAH. They are small, usually measuring between 4 and 7 mm. They originate often on the posterolateral surface of A1 in relation to the origin of perforating arteries. Some A1 aneurysms, however, are of a dissecting nature or originate in context with an A1 fenestration. Suzuki and coworkers [12] classified these aneurysms into five categories according to origin of the aneurysm in relation to the A1 segment: (1) at the junction of the A1 segment and a perforating artery, (2) from the A1 segment directly, (3) from the proximal end of the A1 fenestration, (4) from the junction of the A1 segment and the cortical branch, and (5) fusiform aneurysm.

When planning treatment of an A1 aneurysm, it is important to keep in mind the possibility of a vascular anomaly. It may not be possible to preserve A1 in cases of arterial dissection. In patients whose aneurysms originate from perforating arteries, these perforating arteries are often sacrificed during dissection and clipping. The reported numbers are too small for a final assessment. We have the impression that the morbidity related to perforator injury is minor in comparison with M1 aneurysms.

6.3.2 Dissection and Clipping

These aneurysms are approached the same way as the anterior communicating artery aneurysm. It is important to have a mental picture of the orientation of the aneurysm. In case of the typical perforator-related aneurysm (Fig. 6.13), the dome usually projects upward or posteriorly. The risk of injuring the aneurysm while approaching and dissecting the A1 segment is small.

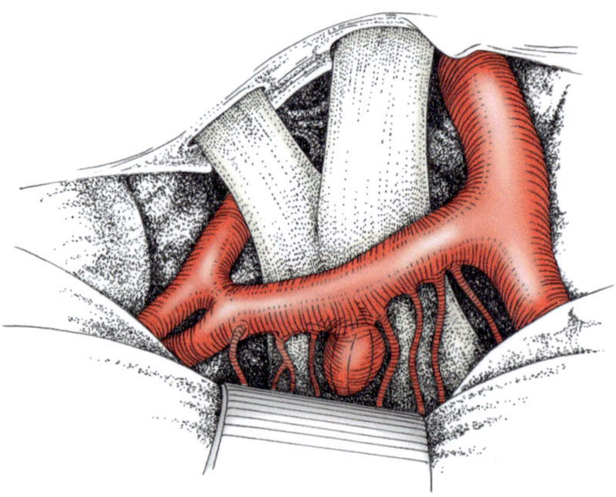

Fig. 6.13 The typical presentation of a perforator-related A1 aneurysm

References

1. Kashimura H, Kubo Y, Ogasawara K, Kakino S, Yoshida K, Ogawa A. Easy dissection of the interhemispheric fissure for treatment of the anterior communicating artery aneurysm by the pterional approach. World Neurosurg. 2010;73:688–90.
2. Suzuki M, Fujisawa H, Ishihara H, Yoneda H, Kato S, Ogawa A. Side selection of pterional approach for anterior communicating artery aneurysms–surgical anatomy and strategy. Acta Neurochir (Wien). 2008;150:31–9.
3. Dengler J, Kato N, Vajkoczy P. The Y-shaped double-barrel bypass in the treatment of large and giant anterior communicating artery aneurysms. J Neurosurg. 2013;118:444–50.
4. Mirzadeh Z, Sanai N, Lawton MT. The azygos anterior cerebral artery bypass: double reimplantation technique for giant anterior communicating artery aneurysms. J Neurosurg. 2011;114:1154–8.
5. Sano H. Treatment of complex intracranial aneurysms of anterior circulation using multiple clips. Acta Neurochir Suppl. 2010;107:27–31.
6. Huber P, Braun J, Hirschmann D, Agyeman JF. Incidence of berry aneurysms of the unpaired pericallosal artery: angiographic study. Neuroradiology. 1980;19:143–7.
7. Perlmutter D, Rhoton Jr AL. Microsurgical anatomy of the distal anterior cerebral artery. J Neurosurg. 1978;49:204–28.
8. Hui FK, Schuette AJ, Moskowitz SI, Spiotta AM, Lieber ML, Rasmussen PA, et al. Microsurgical and endovascular management of pericallosal aneurysms. J Neurointerv Surg. 2011;3:319–23.
9. Kawashima M, Matsushima T, Sasaki T. Surgical strategy for distal anterior cerebral artery aneurysms: microsurgical anatomy. J Neurosurg. 2003;99:517–25.
10. Lehecka M, Dashti R, Lehto H, Kivisaari R, Niemelä M, Hernesniemi J. Distal anterior cerebral artery aneurysms. Acta Neurochir Suppl. 2010;107:15–26.
11. Thomas DG, Paterson A. Results of surgical treatment of pericallosal aneurysms. J Neurol Neurosurg Psychiatry. 1975;38:826.
12. Suzuki M, Onuma T, Sakurai Y, Mizoi K, Ogawa A, Yoshimoto T. Aneurysms arising from the proximal (A1) segment of the anterior cerebral artery. A study of 38 cases. J Neurosurg. 1992;76:455–8.

Suggested Reading

Dashti R, Hernesniemi J, Lehto H, Niemelä M, Lehecka M, Rinne J, et al. Microneurosurgical management of proximal anterior cerebral artery aneurysms. Surg Neurol. 2007;68:366–77.

Hino A, Fujimoto M, Iwamoto Y, Oka H, Echigo T. Surgery of proximal anterior cerebral artery aneurysms. Acta Neurochir (Wien). 2002;144:1291–6; discussion 1296.

Lee JM, Joo SP, Kim TS, Go EJ, Choi HY, Seo BR. Surgical management of anterior cerebral artery aneurysms of the proximal (A1) segment. World Neurosurg. 2010;74:478–82.

Wanibuchi M, Kurokawa Y, Ishiguro M, Fujishige M, Inaba K. Characteristics of aneurysms arising from the horizontal portion of the anterior cerebral artery. Surg Neurol. 2001;55:148–54; discussion 154–5.

Aneurysms of the Middle Cerebral Artery

7

7.1 Aneurysms of the Middle Cerebral Artery Main Bifurcation

7.1.1 General Considerations

Middle cerebral artery (MCA) aneurysms are fairly peripheral to the arterial tree, occurring close to the cranial surface. They are often broad based and rarely lead to a hematoma in the temporal lobe or Sylvian fissure. (Compare also Sect. 7.2.) These factors are in favor of the microsurgical approach, although many MCA aneurysms can technically also be controlled with modern endovascular systems [1, 2].

The location and projection of the aneurysms is important for approach planning. As outlined earlier, we prefer a tailored transsylvian approach in which the M2 segments are identified first and then followed backward to the bifurcation and the neck of the aneurysm.

Planning the approach carefully is important for safe and efficient control of MCA aneurysms. It is important to have a mental concept of the location of the fundus in relation to the bifurcation. The most frequent projections are downward (type 1), with the dome being buried in the temporal lobe (Fig. 7.1), or lateral (type 2), with the aneurysm being more or less a lateral extension of the M1 segment (Fig. 7.2). These latter aneurysms lie in the Sylvian fissure. Type 3 aneurysms lie within the plane of the M2 trunks

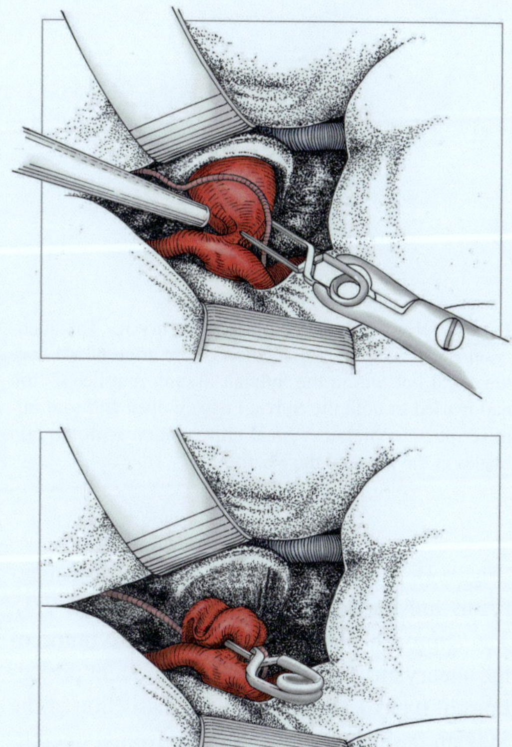

Fig. 7.1 Left-sided type 1 middle cerebral artery (MCA) aneurysm with the dome projecting from the bifurcation toward the temporal lobe. Note the anterior temporal artery curving around the aneurysm. Venous drainage is somewhat atypical in this case in that the main vein runs within the Sylvian fissure. Final clip position following separation of the anterior temporal artery from the aneurysm neck. The plane of the clip is approximately parallel to the plane of the bifurcation

H.-J. Steiger et al., *Microsurgical Brain Aneurysms: Illustrated Concepts and Cases*,
DOI 10.1007/978-3-662-45679-8_7, © Springer-Verlag Berlin Heidelberg 2015

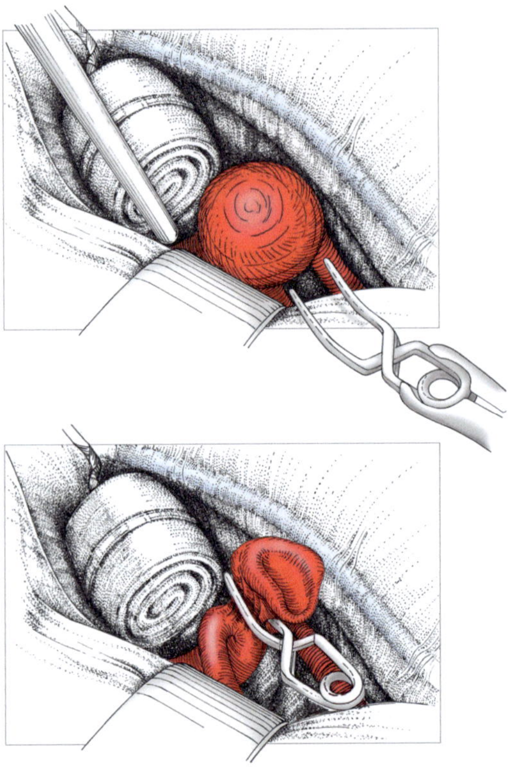

Fig. 7.2 Right-sided type 2 MCA aneurysm. The aneurysm is essentially an elongation of the afferent M1 segment and lies within the Sylvian fissure. A rolled cotton pad is used to hold the Sylvian fissure open and to minimize retractor pressure. Final clip position with the clip blades in the plane of the M2 trunks

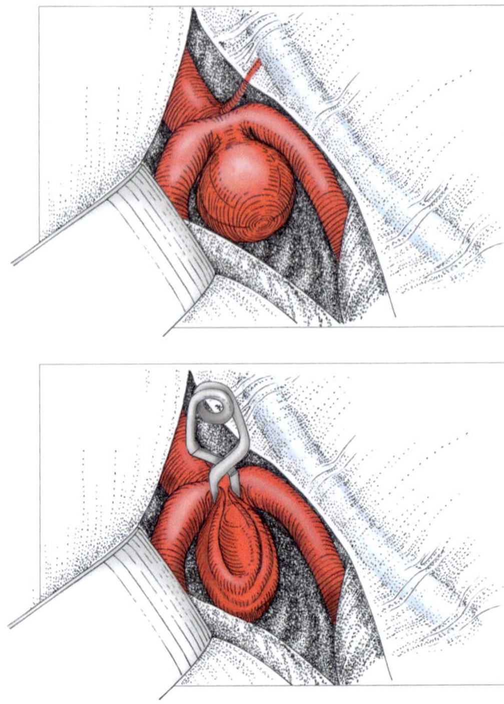

Fig. 7.3 Right-sided type 3 MCA aneurysm. The dome lies between the M2 trunks. Final clip position with the clip perpendicular to the plane of the M2 trunks

(Fig. 7.3). The rare, upward-directed type 4 aneurysms are buried in the frontal lobe (Fig. 7.4). The approach should plan to avoid the dome of the aneurysm. Therefore, for the frequent projections of types 1 and 2, the initial dissection of the Sylvian fissure should follow the frontal operculum down to the superior trunk of the MCA. The position of the dome also must be kept in mind when using retractor blades on the temporal operculum.

The rare frontal projection mandates deviation from the outlined standard strategy. A further exception is the situation of a hematoma in the temporal lobe. Here it is better to proceed through the superior temporal gyrus, as suggested by Heros et al. [3] and Ogilvy et al. [4].

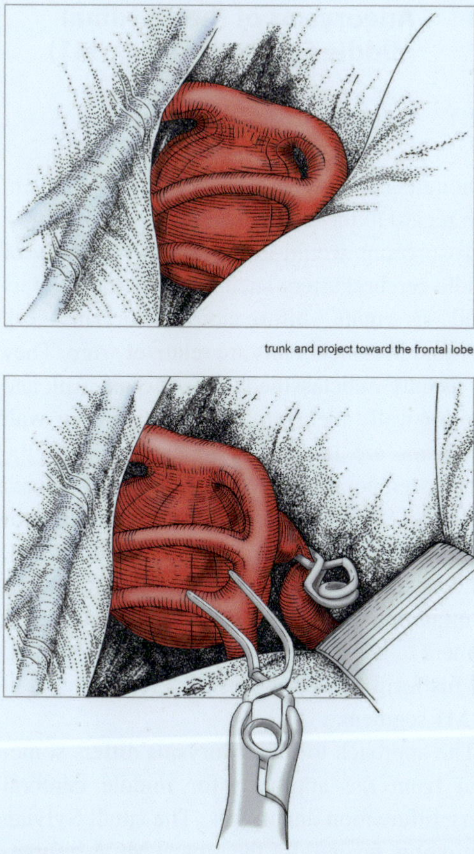

Fig. 7.4 Left-sided type 4 MCA aneurysm. The dome is hidden behind the superior trunk and projects toward the frontal lobe. Following temporary clipping of M1, a curved clip is directed around the superior trunk

7.1.2 Dissection and Clipping

After opening the dura, the Sylvian fissure is subsequently split on the frontal side of the Sylvian vein. One to three venous branches crossing the fissure usually must be coagulated and divided. It is important to split the Sylvian fissure all the way down to the sphenoid ridge to allow for separation of the frontal and temporal lobes. Sufficient dissection at this stage avoids the later necessity to use excessive retraction on the frontal operculum. The superior trunk of the MCA is then identified in the depth of the Sylvian fissure. This artery is then followed proximally to the MCA bifurcation.

To secure proximal control, it is important to keep in mind the course of M1 and the projection of the aneurysm. Most MCA aneurysms are directed more or less toward the temporal lobe. A minority are attached to the frontal side. Therefore proximal control usually is achieved by dissection of the MCA bifurcation along the superior trunk. M1 is identified between the main branches in the case of a high-running M1 segment or in front of the superior trunk in the case of a low-running M1.

Whenever possible, we prefer not to use any brain retractors at all for MCA aneurysms, but sometimes the brain is so swollen that it is impossible to gain sufficient working space without a brain retractor on the frontal operculum. The temporal operculum frequently covers a temporally projecting aneurysm, and it is sometimes necessary to use a small spatula on the temporal operculum during the clipping period.

Temporary clipping of M1 should be used generously whenever the neck of the aneurysm is wider than the diameter of M1. When applying the temporary clip, the origin of the lateral lenticulostriate arteries must be spared.

The final position of the aneurysm clip will be in front of the MCA bifurcation for type 1 projections of the dome and above the bifurcation for type 2. The clip will lie in a plane more or less parallel to the plane of the bifurcation (Fig. 7.1). Dissection of the aneurysm neck is relatively easy with these projections, as the neck is not in direct contact with the M2 trunks.

With type 1 and type 2 aneurysms, however, the anterior temporal artery requires attention. It usually originates on the distal M1 segment and then curves around the aneurysm neck or dome. It must be separated from the neck and spared during clipping. Occlusion of the anterior temporal artery usually leads to infarction of the lateral anterior temporal lobe.

On the other hand, type 3 aneurysms lie between the M2 trunks and need to be separated from these trunks prior to clip application. Here the final clip position will be in a plane more or less perpendicular to the plane of the bifurcation (Fig. 7.3).

The rare upward-projecting aneurysms (type 4) require dissection on the frontal side of the superior MCA main trunk. The lateral lenticulostriate arteries often originate close to the neck of these aneurysms, and particular attention is necessary during dissection and clipping (Fig. 7.5).

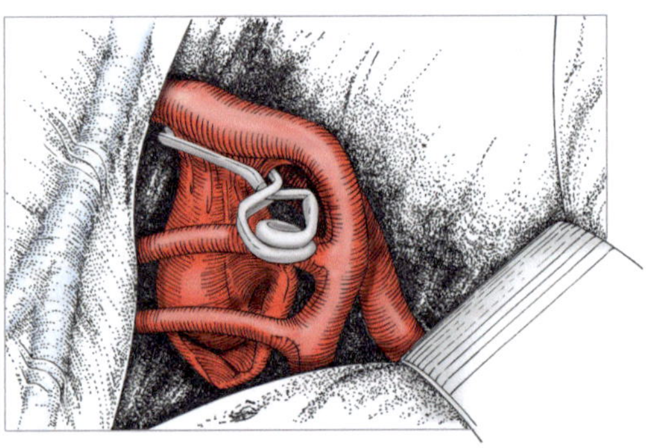

Fig. 7.5 Final clip position for type 4 with the clip parallel to the plane of the M2 trunks. Particular attention must be paid to the lenticulostriate arteries, which are often close to the neck of type 4 aneurysms (*not shown*)

7.2 Aneurysms of the Proximal Middle Cerebral Artery (M1)

7.2.1 General Considerations

Although there is considerable disagreement with regard to the anatomical classification, most neurosurgeons would agree that the majority of middle cerebral artery aneurysms should be classified as main bifurcation aneurysms [5]. Proximal M1 aneurysms are relatively rare. They are usually subclassified into inferior-wall and superior-wall aneurysms [6, 7]. Inferior-wall aneurysms are in relation to the origin of the anterior temporal artery or a frontal M1 branch (Fig. 7.6). Superior-wall aneurysms have a topographical relation to the lenticulostriate arteries, and these aneurysms carry a risk of lenticulostriate infarction with clipping. As with the proximal segment of the anterior cerebral artery, dissecting and fusiform aneurysms also are rarely found at the M1 segment.

The approach to M1 aneurysms differs somewhat from the approach for middle cerebral artery bifurcation aneurysms. The small Sylvian craniotomy favored for the typical MCA bifurcation aneurysm has no advantage over the pterional craniotomy for M1 aneurysms and may be even more awkward. Exposure is more challenging than for the bifurcation aneurysm, because the surgeon needs to maneuver around the main bifurcation for dissection and clip application. When using the Sylvian craniotomy, it is important to split the Sylvian fissure proximally down to the sphenoid ridge in order to obtain sufficient space.

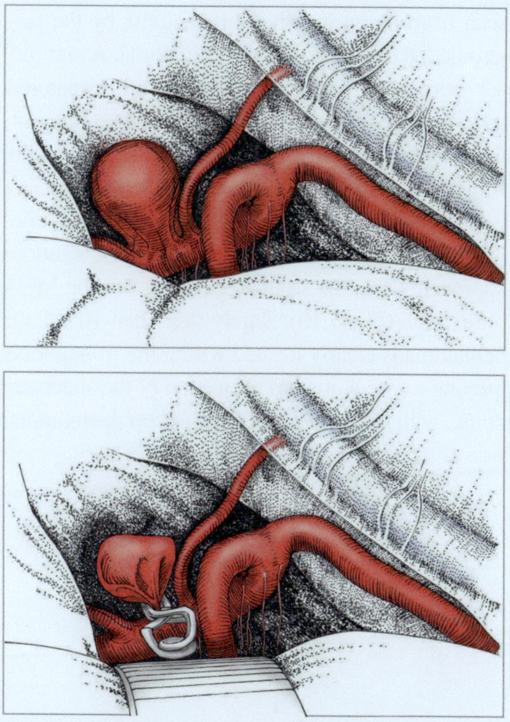

Fig. 7.6 Inferior-wall aneurysm of the right M1 between a frontal branch and the anterior temporal artery. Final clip position

7.2.2 Dissection and Clipping

Dissection and clipping of an inferior-wall aneurysm is straightforward. Dissection involves separation of the proximal branching artery from the neck, i.e., the anterior temporal artery.

Superior-wall aneurysms are tricky to expose. Furthermore, dissection of the adjacent lenticulostriate arteries is difficult, particularly because the aneurysms are often relatively broad based and incorporate the origin of a lenticulostriate branch. The same applies to clipping. The potential compromise of lenticulostriate arteries mandates careful verification of patency following clip application. Micro-Doppler and indocyanine green (ICG) angiography are not without limitation in this situation, owing to the narrow and relatively deep surgical field.

7.3 Middle Cerebral Artery Aneurysm with Intracerebral Mass Hemorrhage

7.3.1 Specific Clinical Considerations

Approximately one third of ruptured MCA aneurysms present with acute intracerebral hemorrhage. Because of the temporal position of the hematoma and the additional subarachnoid blood component, relatively small hematomas lead to critical mass effect with midline shift and resulting depression of the level of consciousness [8]. Hemorrhage volumes of more than 20 mL should be considered critical. The indication for emergency evacuation must be based on the patient's clinical condition as well as the volume of the hematoma. MCA aneurysms leading to intracerebral hemorrhage are generally larger than the average MCA aneurysm, most often between 10 and 15 mm. Very rarely, small aneurysms are the source of an intracerebral hemorrhage. Previous subarachnoid hemorrhage (SAH) leading to adhesion between the aneurysm and pia mater is considered a plausible explanation for intracerebral hemorrhage with small aneurysms. Poor-grade patients with intracerebral temporal hemorrhage often recover surprisingly well after evacuation of the hematoma and securing of the aneurysms, but patients with Sylvian hematomas often suffer pronounced delayed ischemia and overall have a relatively poor outcome [9, 10].

7.3.2 Preoperative Work-Up and Microsurgical Indication

Evacuation of mass hemorrhage and elimination of the aneurysm is time critical. The usual work-up with angiography after SAH often cannot be applied without further compromising the patient's neurological condition and chances of recovery. Therefore, it is our practice to limit the presurgical work-up in stuporous or comatose patients to the plain CT, which provides the essential information required for surgery: the location of the hematoma (temporal, Sylvian, or frontal) provides the necessary information regarding the projection of the aneurysm dome in relation to the MCA bifurcation. The hematoma is located in the temporal lobe in approximately 60 % of cases, proving a type 1 projection with the dome toward the temporal lobe (Figs. 7.7 and 7.8). M1 and the origin of both M2 trunks are on the frontal side of the aneurysm, within the Sylvian fissure. In contrast, the hematoma lies completely or largely within the Sylvian fissure in approximately 20–30 % of cases. A Sylvian hematoma can be distinguished on the CT scan from an intratemporal hematoma by the posteromedial delineation of the hematoma. A curvilinear border suggests an intratemporal hematoma, whereas wavy posteromedial delineation suggests that the hematoma lies intrasylvian (curtain sign) (Fig. 7.9). A Sylvian hematoma proves a type 2 or type 3 projection of the aneurysm; i.e., the dome lies within the Sylvian fissure, requiring a cautious approach along the frontal operculum to the MCA bifurcation (Fig. 7.10). Rarely (less than 10 %), the hematoma is clearly located within the frontal lobe, proving a type 4 upward projection of the aneurysm dome, with both M2 trunks located on the temporal side of the aneurysm.

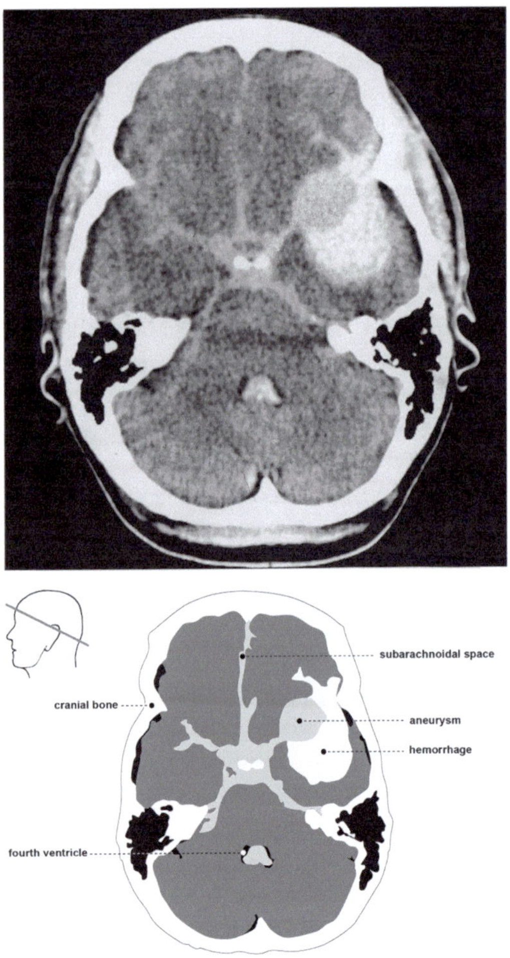

Fig. 7.7 Typical case of mass hemorrhage in the left temporal pole, suggesting a type 1 aneurysm projection

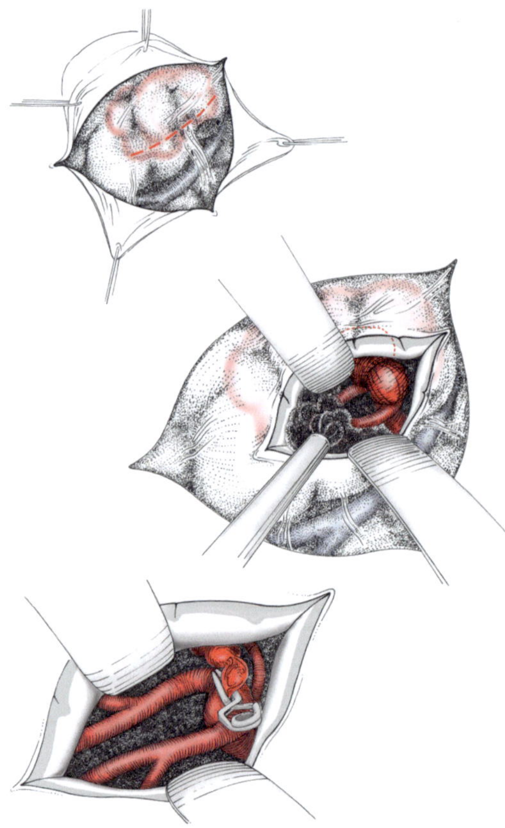

Fig. 7.8 The hematoma is accessed through the superior temporal gyrus and carefully decompressed. Following control of the bifurcation, the clip is applied above the M2 trunks

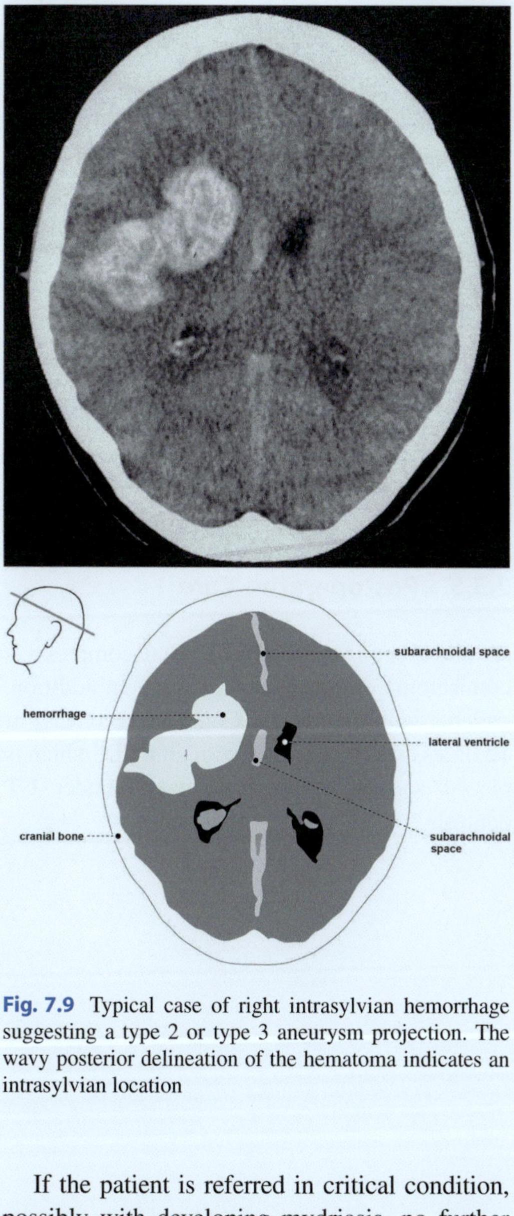

Fig. 7.9 Typical case of right intrasylvian hemorrhage suggesting a type 2 or type 3 aneurysm projection. The wavy posterior delineation of the hematoma indicates an intrasylvian location

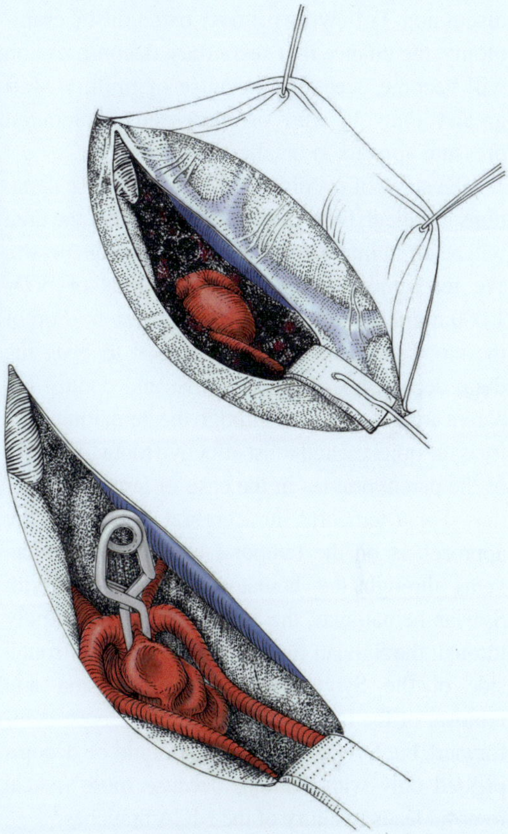

Fig. 7.10 The Sylvian fissure is opened on the frontal side of the Sylvian vein and the hematoma is carefully decompressed. Here the aneurysm has a type 3 projection and is located between the M2 trunks. The clip direction is typically perpendicular to the plane of the bifurcation

If the patient is referred in critical condition, possibly with developing mydriasis, no further diagnostic procedures beyond plain CT should be done; the patient should be directed straight to the OR. We recommend giving 50–100 g mannitol in patients with developing mydriasis. On the other hand, if CT diagnostics are done after admission in the neurosurgical department, adding a CT angiography sequence in addition to the plain CT scan is certainly useful.

7.3.3 Positioning and Approach

The shoulder should be supported by a cushion and the head should be rotated 60° contralaterally. We do not recommend insertion of an external ventricular drain (EVD) prior to evacuation of the hematoma, and use of spinal drainage is contraindicated. We recommend planning for decompressive craniectomy in the case of comatose patients, but this advice is a matter of recurring discussion. Following primary osteoplastic craniotomy, the chance that secondary decompression will become necessary because of midline shift greater than 10 mm or increased intracranial pressure appears to be about 50 %.

The stage of opening of the dura in these situations is critical. If the dura is tense, opening the dura will result in immediate rerupture of the aneurysm. We recommend administering a bolus of 500–1,000 mg thiopental, leading to a transient drop of the blood pressure; this time is used to open the dura, decompress the hematoma, and control the parent arteries. The way through the hematoma cavity is the quickest and most effective route to control of the parent arteries in the case of larger hematomas. For a temporal intracerebral hematoma, the approach is on the temporal side of the Sylvian veins through the hematoma cavity [4]. With Sylvian hematomas, the best approach is naturally through the Sylvian fissure, which is on the frontal side of the Sylvian vein. Decompression and removal of the intracerebral hematoma is straightforward, but Sylvian hematomas should be decompressed only with caution, because more radical removal leads to injury of the MCA branches.

7.3.4 Dissection and Clipping

Following control of M1, the aneurysm neck is dissected and the M2 trunks are identified. With the most common type of projection, the clip direction is from the frontal side to the temporal side over the bifurcation, and the clip plane is parallel to the plane of the bifurcation. With type 1 or 2 projection of the aneurysmal dome associated with temporal or Sylvian hematoma, the direction of the clip is above and parallel to the plane of the M2 segments (Fig. 7.8). With type 3 aneurysms, the clip direction is perpendicular to the plane of the bifurcation, with the branches passing between the M2 trunks (Fig. 7.10).

7.3.5 Postoperative Care

As mentioned, we recommend decompressive craniectomy for comatose patients. In addition, patients with a Glasgow Coma Score (GCS) of 12 or less should be fitted with an EVD, which is placed some 6 h postoperatively, under CT control.

References

1. Brinjikji W, Lanzino G, Cloft HJ, Rabinstein A, Kallmes DF. Endovascular treatment of middle cerebral artery aneurysms: a systematic review and single-center series. Neurosurgery. 2011;68:397–402.
2. Rodríguez-Hernández A, Sughrue ME, Akhavan S, Habdank-Kolaczkowski J, Lawton MT. Current management of middle cerebral artery aneurysms: surgical results with a "clip first" policy. Neurosurgery. 2013;72:415–27.
3. Heros RC, Ojemann RG, Crowell RM. Superior temporal gyrus approach to middle cerebral artery aneurysms: technique and results. Neurosurgery. 1982;10:308–13.
4. Ogilvy CS, Crowell RM, Heros RC. Surgical management of middle cerebral artery aneurysms: experience with transsylvian and superior temporal gyrus approaches. Surg Neurol. 1995;43:15–22; discussion 22–4.
5. Ulm AJ, Fautheree GL, Tanriover N, Russo A, Albanese E, Rhoton Jr AL, et al. Microsurgical and angiographic anatomy of middle cerebral artery aneurysms: prevalence and significance of early branch aneurysms. Neurosurgery. 2008;62(5 Suppl 2): ONS344–52.
6. Ha SK, Lim DJ, Kang SH, Kim SH, Park JY, Chung YG. Analysis of multiple factors affecting surgical outcomes of proximal middle cerebral artery aneurysms. Clin Neurol Neurosurg. 2011;113:362–7.
7. Paulo MS, Edgardo S, Fernando M, Pablo P, Alejandro T, Verónica V. Aneurysms of the middle cerebral artery proximal segment (M1). Anatomical and therapeutic considerations. Revision of a series. Analysis of a series of the pre bifurcation segment aneurysms. Asian J Neurosurg. 2010;5:57–63.
8. Tapaninaho A, Hernesniemi J, Vapalahti M. Emergency treatment of cerebral aneurysms with large haematomas. Acta Neurochir (Wien). 1988; 91:21–4.
9. Otani N, Takasato Y, Masaoka H, Hayakawa T, Yoshino Y, Yatsushige H, et al. Surgical outcome following decompressive craniectomy for poor-grade aneurysmal subarachnoid hemorrhage in patients with associated massive intracerebral or Sylvian hematomas. Cerebrovasc Dis. 2008;26:612–7.
10. Bohnstedt BN, Nguyen HS, Kulwin CG, Shoja MM, Helbig GM, Leipzig TJ, et al. Outcomes for clip ligation and hematoma evacuation associated with 102 patients with ruptured middle cerebral artery aneurysms. World Neurosurg. 2013;80:335–41.

8 Aneurysms of the Internal Carotid Artery

Aneurysms of the internal carotid artery (ICA) are subdivided according to their location along the ICA into proximal or paraclinoid aneurysms, aneurysms of the middle segment, and terminal aneurysms. Aneurysms may be related to branches of the ICA—that is, the ophthalmic artery, the posterior communicating artery (Pcom), or the anterior choroidal artery (AChA)—but a considerable proportion are unrelated to side branches. Aneurysms of the ICA can reach giant size and present with optic nerve compression.

Very small, blister-like aneurysms that present with subarachnoid hemorrhage (SAH) typically also occur on the ICA. Although surgical management using wrapping techniques is possible, the trend in the literature indicates a clear shift toward endovascular management of blister-like ICA aneurysms using stents or flow diverters, so these aneurysms are not considered in this chapter.

Saccular ICA aneurysms presenting with SAH should be treated by the endovascular route if that is considered feasible, in light of the neck configuration. The best treatment for large aneurysms leading to optic nerve compression, or third nerve palsy in the case of the ICA-Pcom aneurysm, is a matter of debate. Microsurgical clipping leads to immediate relief of the compression, thus creating optimal conditions for recovery. On the other hand, a significant rate of recovery from both vision loss and third nerve palsy is reported following endovascular treatment. Nevertheless, the use of endovascular tools to manage large and giant aneurysms is still disappointing with regard to early complication rates and long-term stability. At this time, we recommend microsurgical obliteration as first choice, if the specific anatomy of the aneurysm appears favorable for exposure and clip elimination.

H.-J. Steiger et al., *Microsurgical Brain Aneurysms: Illustrated Concepts and Cases*,
DOI 10.1007/978-3-662-45679-8_8, © Springer-Verlag Berlin Heidelberg 2015

8.1 ICA–Ophthalmic Artery Aneurysms

8.1.1 General Considerations

ICA–ophthalmic artery aneurysms are the most frequent and clinically most important subtype of the paraclinoid aneurysms. They are located dorsally on the ICA and project toward the optic nerve. They present either with unilateral visual loss or with SAH. Aneurysms presenting with optic nerve compression usually have considerable size, which translates to specific challenges for the microsurgical approach.

The ophthalmic artery originates from the intradural segment of the ICA in over 90 % of individuals. Nonetheless, complete visualization of the base of the aneurysm and in particular of the ophthalmic artery requires extensive dissection with removal of the anterior clinoid process. Because extensive bone removal is associated with additional risk, we do not recommend its general and uncritical use. Some ICA–ophthalmic artery aneurysms are partially located in the cavernous sinus. Postoperative neck remnants in the cavernous sinus usually can be treated well via the endovascular route, and it appears not to be justified to extend intraoperative dissection into the cavernous sinus.

ICA–ophthalmic artery aneurysms present a unique challenge: proximal control is not available during dissection and clipping. Proximal control is important not only to control bleeding in case of intraoperative aneurysm rupture but also to reduce intra-aneurysmal pressure during clip application. Reducing intra-aneurysmal pressure during clip application is essential with large ICA–ophthalmic artery aneurysms; otherwise, they will tear at the base when the clip is applied.

An obvious solution could be to control the extracranial internal carotid artery at the neck by a separate surgical exposure or by the endovascular route with the help of a balloon catheter; but blocking the proximal ICA alone does not help much, as retrograde flow through the ophthalmic artery cannot be controlled in this way. The arterial collateralization of the face is so rich that occlusion of the cervical external carotid artery is useless. Batjer and colleagues [1] developed the so-called retrograde suction decompression technique to cope with the problem (compare Fig. 8.1). Through a catheter inserted in the cervical carotid artery, blood is aspirated during clip application. Today this can be achieved effectively via the endovascular route if intraoperative angiography or a hybrid operating suite is available.

Alternatives to the suction decompression method to render the aneurysm supple during clip application include temporary deep hypotension or short-term cardiac arrest using adenosine [2, 3]. These methods are simpler than retrograde suction decompression and complications are rare if they are used correctly (mainly by limiting the duration to a few minutes). Normotensive and otherwise healthy patients tolerate well induced hypotension to a mean arterial pressure of 40 mmHg for a maximum of 5 min. We recommend the use of induced hypotension if the aneurysm has a clearly delineated neck with preservation of the contour of the parent artery; we reserve retrograde suction decompression for broad-based aneurysms with inclusion of the ICA wall.

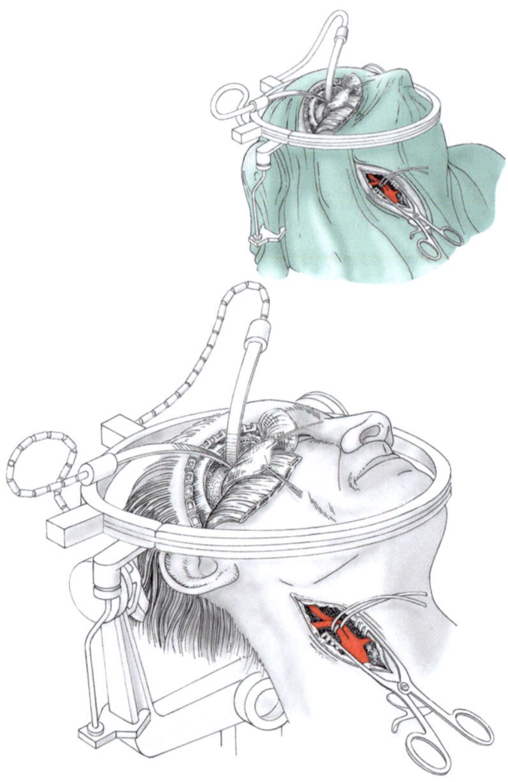

Fig. 8.1 Simultaneous craniotomy and exposure of the cervical carotid bifurcation for complex paraophthalmic aneurysms (OR setting). Details of the simultaneous approach to cranial and cervical exposure for complex paraophthalmic aneurysms

8.1.2 Dissection of ICA–Ophthalmic Artery Aneurysm and Clipping

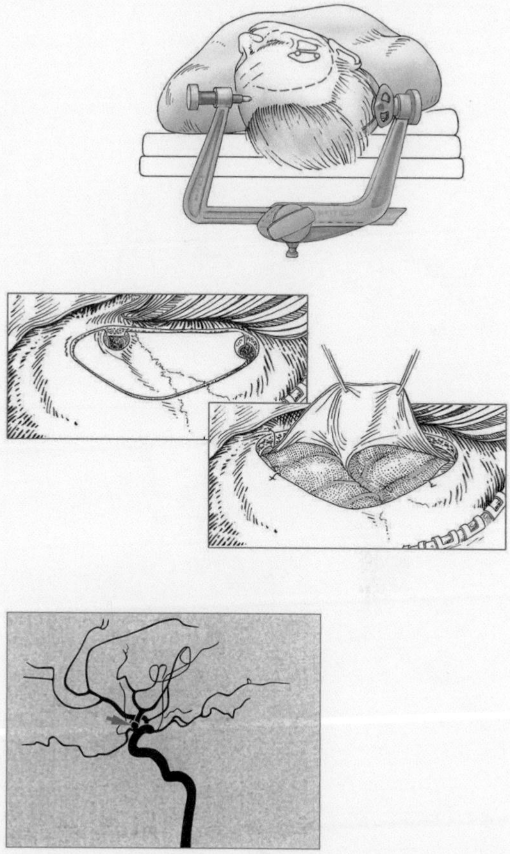

Fig. 8.2 Custom-tailored pterional craniotomy: head positioning, skin incision (*broken line*), craniotomy (*continuous line*). Dural opening. Digital subtraction angiography showing aneurysm (*arrow*)

A custom-tailored pterional craniotomy as described in detail in Chap. 4 (Fig. 8.2) is used for the approach. The head is positioned with an approximately 45-degree rotation to the contralateral side and slightly hyperextended. A spinal drain is inserted in case of recent SAH, unless ventriculostomy has been placed on the basis of a World Federation of Neurosurgical Societies (WFNS) grade of 4 or worse.

Before opening the dura, sufficient brain relaxation is achieved by drainage of 50–100 mL of CSF, in case of SAH, and by mannitol if necessary (1–2 g/kg body weight). Because a larger aneurysm requires a large working space, the Sylvian fissure should be completely opened from the periphery down to the clinoid, to allow mobilization of the frontal and orbital cortex without applying undue pressure with a retractor blade. Care needs to be taken not to tear the aneurysm when opening the carotid cistern. For smaller aneurysms, splitting the fissure may be limited to the central aspect. Following gentle elevation of the orbital cortex, the proximal carotid artery and the optic nerve are identified. The optic nerve and the carotid artery are freed of arachnoid adhesions and the prechiasmatic cistern is opened. The distal delineation of the aneurysm neck comes in view at this point. Further dissection of the aneurysm neck clarifies whether removal of the anterior clinoid process becomes necessary. If the dissector can be passed proximally underneath the clinoid over the carotid, removal is not necessary. Otherwise, the anterior clinoid is gently drilled with a diamond drill and the optic nerve is unroofed by splitting the falciform ligament. This maneuver provides some additional space and allows visualization of the ICA down to the entry point into the cavernous sinus. Dissection of the aneurysm neck is completed now on the proximal side beneath the clinoid and the optic foramen. Because the aneurysm obscures vision, the back side usually cannot be seen completely. Dissection is complete when the tip of the dissector reaches bone.

At that time, decisions must be made with regard to making the aneurysm supple for clip application and with regard to the clip technique. If the neck is relatively narrow, short-term induced hypotension is appropriate, and a straight clip can be passed over the top of the ICA. As an alternative, sequential clipping with a palisade of small clips can be used (Fig. 8.3).

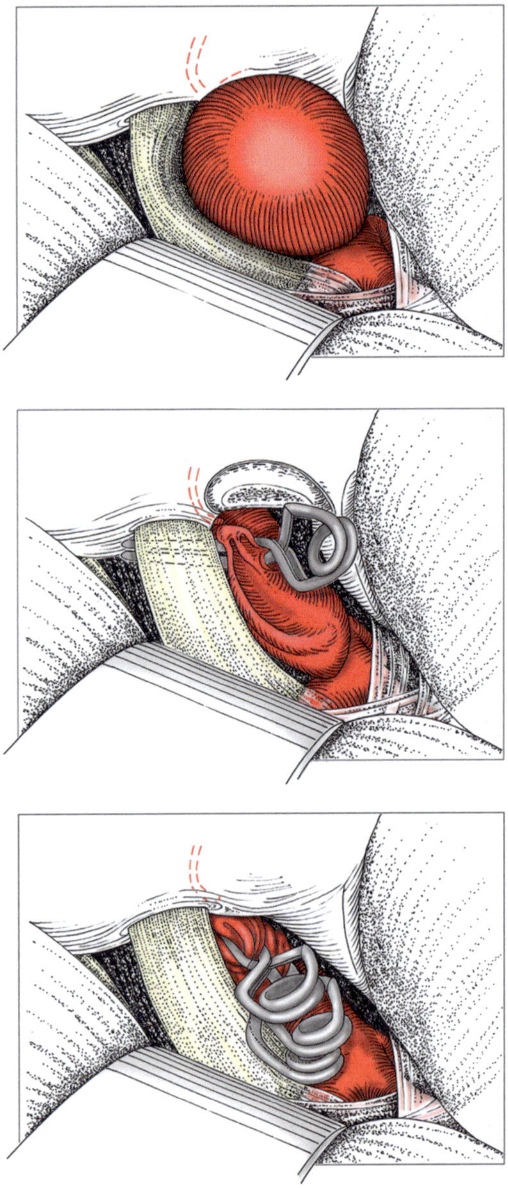

Fig. 8.3 Paraophthalmic aneurysm showing compression of the optic nerve and the presumed course of the ophthalmic artery. Horizontal clip positioning (variant a). Stepwise vertical clipping with multiple clips (variant b)

ICA–ophthalmic artery aneurysms differ from other aneurysms also with regard to temporary clipping if proximal control can be obtained beneath the clinoid. If a sufficient segment of proximal ICA is available, proximal temporary clipping should be done. The effect of proximal ICA clipping on the intra-aneurysmal pressure varies considerably, however, owing to retrograde flow from the distal ICA and the ophthalmic artery. The usual response to insufficient aneurysm relaxation following clipping of the proximal parent artery is additional distal clipping to block retrograde flow, but in the case of an ICA–ophthalmic artery aneurysm, the usual result of distal clipping is an increase in intra-aneurysmal pressure because residual inflow comes from the ophthalmic artery, and applying a temporary clip on the distal ICA blocks the outflow and raises the intra-aneurysmal pressure again to systemic arterial pressure. Therefore, the effect of proximal temporary clipping on intra-aneurysmal turgor must be watched carefully. If it is unsatisfactory, improvement can be expected only from systemic hypotension or other measures as discussed above.

8.1.3 Special Aspects

The retrograde suction decompression method, open or via the endovascular route, is generally accepted for giant and broad-based aneurysms. Although this maneuver is definitely helpful, it is by no means the cure for all problems and is associated with its own specific complications, such as thromboembolism. We prefer systemic hypotension, except with giant aneurysms. We developed a special balloon-assisted method (further discussed in Chap. 10) to temporarily occlude the aneurysm neck, but experience to date is not yet sufficient for a final assessment of its benefits and risks.

8.2 ICA–Posterior Communicating Artery Aneurysms

8.2.1 General Considerations

Today, patients with Pcom aneurysms are considered candidates primarily for microsurgery if they have hematomas, recurrent aneurysms after coiling, Pcom arising from the aneurysm neck, aneurysms causing oculomotor nerve palsy, or multiple aneurysms.

In principle, aneurysms at the ICA-Pcom position are straightforward. Exposure does not provide major challenges, as the approach path is naturally quite wide. There is no need for skull base drilling or significant brain retraction. Proximal control is easy to obtain, and clip application is not critical, as there are no critical perforators in the immediate vicinity. These initial impressions are counterbalanced, however, by their relatively proximal location on the vascular tree. If the parent artery cannot be preserved, ischemic damage is often major, depending on the collateral flow. In the worst case, hemispheric infarction can result from failed surgery.

A few points require particular attention, and some pitfalls must be avoided. The Pcom occasionally has a very proximal origin, with resulting difficulty in obtaining proximal control. It may be necessary in some cases to drill the anterior clinoid process in order to expose the proximal ICA. A further difficulty arises from broad-necked aneurysms that incorporate the origin of the Pcom. This artery should be preserved by all means; preservation is critical when the Pcom has a large diameter—that is, when it is supplying the posterior cerebral artery. In the case of a large Pcom, the hypothalamic and mesencephalic perforators arising from this artery originate on the ICA side of the Pcom, and occlusion of the Pcom origin at the ICA also leads to occlusion or thrombosis of these critical perforators, with subsequent hemiparesis.

A further particularity of the ICA-Pcom aneurysm relates to the age distribution of the patients. On one hand, ICA-Pcom aneurysms represent a preferential location in young patients. It appears that in young patients, these aneurysms have a relatively high rate of recurrence if not perfectly eliminated. Therefore it is important to strive for a perfect solution, using a curved clip to optimally match the curvature of the ICA. On the other hand, the ICA-Pcom location is also a preferential aneurysm site in elderly women. In this group particularly, the aneurysm neck is often wide, and the Pcom occasionally arises from the neck. In this situation, it is often necessary to leave a small part of the aneurysm open in the form of an infundibulum for the Pcom. This is achieved best by using a straight clip that imperfectly matches the curvature of the carotid wall. In our experience, this residual dog-ear does not translate to the risk of aneurysm recurrence in elderly patients.

8.2.2 Dissection and Clipping

Presurgical preparation, anesthesia, and positioning are equivalent to those for an ICA–ophthalmic artery aneurysm. A small pterional craniotomy also is well suited for these aneurysms. The head is positioned with an approximately 45-degree rotation to the contralateral side and is slightly hyperextended.

Splitting the Sylvian fissure should be done according to the specific needs. Elongation of the ICA in elderly patients makes complete opening of the fissure often necessary in order to gain sufficient exposure. In contrast, it is not necessary to split the fissure completely in the case of a proximally located aneurysm; it is enough to split the central aspect of the fissure and the carotid cistern. Following gentle elevation of the orbital cortex, the proximal carotid artery and the optic nerve are identified and freed of arachnoid adhesions. In the case of an elongated ICA with subsequent posterior and upward displacement of the aneurysm, it may be necessary to use a second spatula for gentle posterior retraction of the temporal pole. In contrast to middle cerebral artery aneurysms, the use of one or two spatulas is most often helpful and necessary (Fig. 8.4).

The distal delineation of the aneurysm neck usually comes in view first. The angle between the aneurysm neck and the distal ICA is dissected. The origin of the anterior choroidal artery (AChA) is usually separated from the neck by some millimeters and is not in danger during dissection of the typical Pcom aneurysm. Further dissection of the aneurysm neck identifies the proximal neck and here in particular the relation to the Pcom that originates on the back wall of the ICA and then turns medially. The origin of the artery is usually identified by dissection lateral to the ICA and its further course medial between the ICA and the optic chiasm. It is important to keep the third nerve in mind during further dissection, with the aneurysm beneath the tentorial edge. Further dissection must clarify how far the proximal neck can be separated from the Pcom origin.

As mentioned, with very proximally located or large Pcom aneurysms, it is sometimes necessary also to drill the anterior clinoid process with a diamond drill and unroof the optic nerve to gain proximal control.

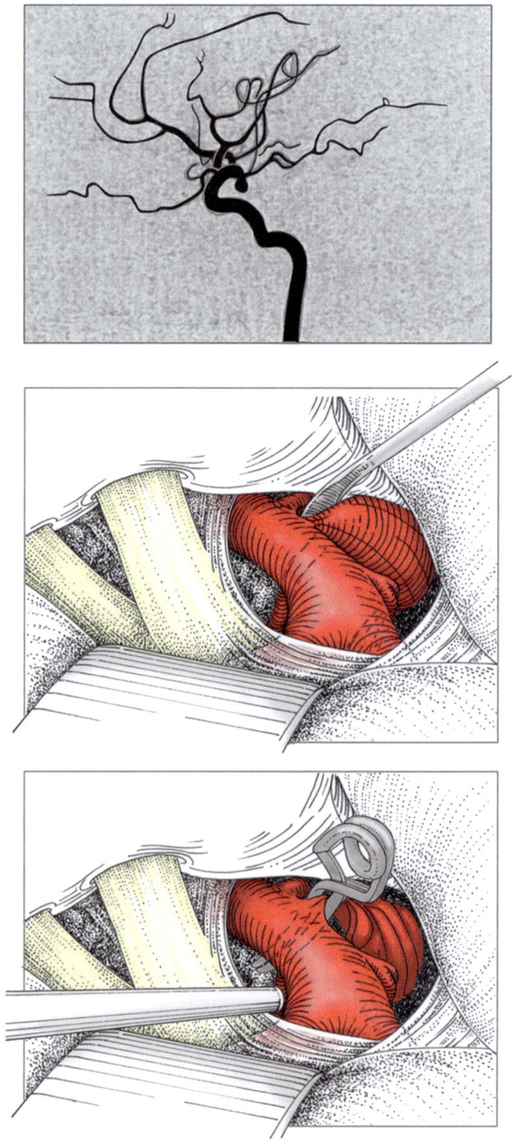

Fig. 8.4 Digital subtraction angiography showing a posterior communicating artery (Pcom) aneurysm. Dissecting the aneurysm base carefully from the Pcom and the anterior choroidal artery (AChA). Application of a curved clip to achieve an optimal reconstruction

Following complete dissection, a decision must be made about the mode of clipping. If the Pcom can be separated from the neck down to the ICA, a perfect solution using a curved clip should be aimed for. On the other hand, if complete separation of the Pcom origin is not possible, an imperfect solution using a straight clip should be opted for, which leaves a small dog-ear as an infundibulum of the Pcom.

Temporary clipping of the proximal ICA is recommended with all broad-based aneurysms. That is, we recommend temporary clipping whenever the diameter of the neck is larger than the diameter of the ICA.

8.2.3 Additional Remarks

As Sanai and coworkers [4] pointed out recently, the microsurgical spectrum of ICA-Pcom aneurysms changed considerably after the introduction of endovascular therapy. The current mix of Pcom aneurysms occasionally requires advanced techniques including clinoidectomy, AChA microdissection, and complex clip reconstruction, which were seldom necessary for the treatment of Pcom aneurysms prior to the introduction of endovascular therapy.

8.3 ICA–Anterior Choroidal Artery Aneurysms

8.3.1 General Considerations

Aneurysms of anterior choroidal artery (AChA) origin make up 2–4 % of all ruptured and unruptured aneurysms. They are usually rather small and become symptomatic with SAH or, rarely, epilepsy. Unruptured AChA aneurysms are often detected in a setting of multiple aneurysms. The AChA is a terminal perforator supplying part of the internal capsule. Occlusion of the AChA invariably results in hemiparesis. Surgical results for AChA aneurysms have previously been reported as unsatisfactory owing to inadvertent occlusion of the AChA, and ischemic complications with resulting hemiparesis have been reported as high as 25 % [5]. The risk of AChA occlusion can be minimized by taking every precaution to preserve AChA patency and also by using intraoperative monitoring that will alert the surgeon to AChA compromise. Assessing patency with the help of micro-Doppler and indocyanine green (ICG) angiography is also particularly critical for aneurysms in this location.

8.3.2 Approach and Clipping

The approach is straightforward and comparable to the approach for the ICA-Pcom aneurysm. The ICA is exposed and dissected distally up to the bifurcation, so sufficient opening of the Sylvian fissure is mandatory.

Dissection of the AChA from the neck is critical, and time should be taken for this step. We recommend the use of intraoperative irrigation with nimodipine solution for all aneurysms, but its use may be particularly important to prevent spasm in the case of AChA dissection. The AChA may arise occasionally from the neck of the aneurysm, which compromises a perfect clipping solution. In this situation, a small remnant of the aneurysm must be left in order to protect AChA inflow.

If possible, application of a curved clip should be preferred because this configuration allows perfect reconstruction of the carotid contour (Fig. 8.5).

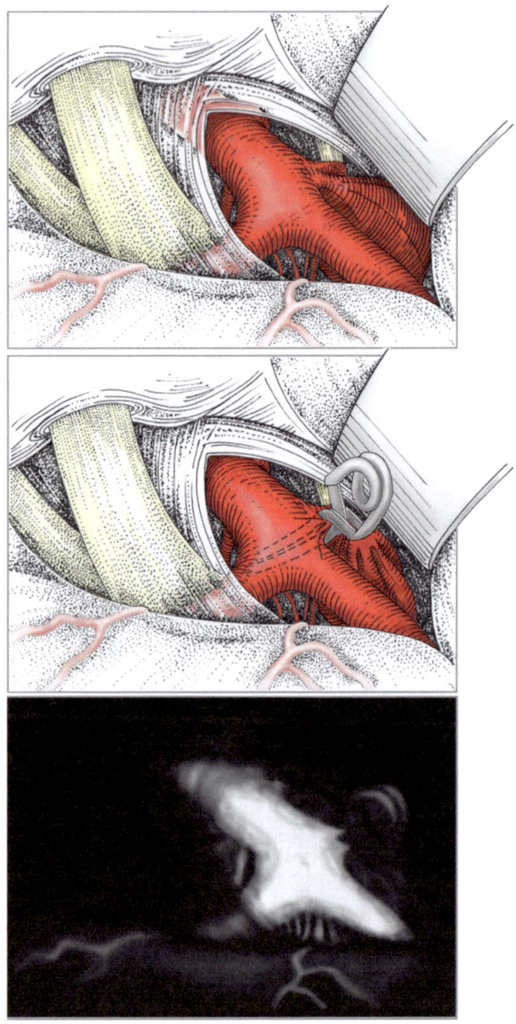

Fig. 8.5 Typical ICA–anterior choroidal artery (AChA) aneurysm. Clip positioning (curved clip recommended). Indocyanine green (ICG) video angiography to confirm AChA patency after clip positioning

8.4 Giant Aneurysms of the Anterior and Posterior Walls

8.4.1 General Considerations

Giant aneurysms of the anterior and posterior walls are considered to originate independent of a side branch, as a result of some ill-defined vasculopathy. They most often become symptomatic with signs of compression, headache, or ischemic symptoms. These aneurysms are rare and treatment is problematic because of the underlying vascular dysplasia. It is difficult to reconstruct an anatomically normal vascular contour. Clipping may result in straightening and elongation of the segment with consequent kinking of the adjacent distal carotid segment and the anterior and middle cerebral artery.

Sugita and coworkers [6, 7] introduced stepwise reconstruction with multiple clips and developed angled, fenestrated clips to reconstruct fusiform posterior wall aneurysms. Yasargil [8] preferred the use of straight clips passed behind the carotid artery. Anterior aneurysms are generally clipped with a palisade of straight clips.

The principal long-term problem with these aneurysms is related to the underlying vascular dysplasia. The aneurysms have a tendency to recur or regrow because the residual wall consists mainly of immature collagen and is largely devoid of a normal tunica media with smooth muscle cells. Furthermore, in order to prevent stenosis, vascular reconstruction aims to reach a wider vascular diameter rather than one that is too narrow. The rate of secondary regrowth is thus substantial, although exact numbers are unavailable because of the small number of these aneurysms.

If these aneurysms recur, permanent cure can be achieved by endovascular occlusion of the affected vascular segment, if collateral circulation is sufficient. To optimize preconditions for later occlusive treatment, we recommend combining the initial procedure with an extracranial–intracranial (EC–IC) bypass. This maneuver may provide some protection during prolonged ischemia, but it mainly will be used if occlusive therapy should later become necessary [9].

8.4.2 Exposure and Clipping

A standard pterional approach is favored for these aneurysms. Generous splitting of the Sylvian fissure is mandatory for a safe working space. The aneurysm comes immediately into view when opening the fissure. Gaining proximal control is usually easily possible with posterior wall aneurysms (i.e., when the normal anterior wall is encountered first). It may be necessary to drill off the anterior clinoid process in order to define the proximal end of the aneurysm and gain proximal control.

Exposure of the proximal ICA may be more difficult with anterior wall aneurysms, where the aneurysm is in the way to the proximal ICA (Fig. 8.6).

If an EC–IC bypass is planned, it should be done in a standard fashion at the beginning of the operation. It is important to perform a standard superficial temporal artery to middle cerebral artery branch bypass. The use of venous or radial

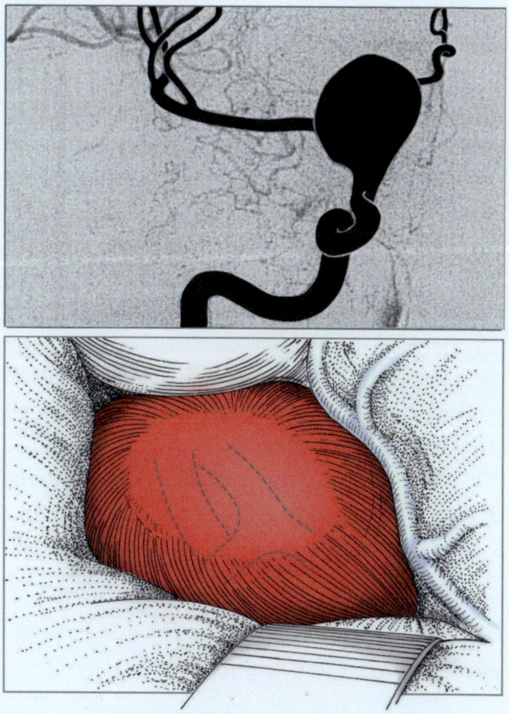

Fig. 8.6 Digital subtraction angiography showing giant ICA anterior wall aneurysm. Operative view following opening the Sylvian fissure

grafts must be avoided because these grafts will thrombose if not perfused sufficiently. Standard EC–IC anastomoses usually remain patent even if there is no need for additional flow, and they can resume function years later if need occurs.

Dissection and preservation of the AChA is critical, particularly with posterior wall aneurysms. Most often the AChA arises distal to the aneurysm, close to the bifurcation. The artery is usually stretched over the lateral aspect of the aneurysm dome and is quite adherent. It is well worth taking some time to dissect it off over the entire distance of adherence to the dome.

Prior to clipping the aneurysm, it is important to achieve softening of the aneurysm by proximal temporary clipping and possibly additional induced hypotension, as with the ICA–ophthalmic artery aneurysm. Temporary trapping may be useful in case of a small Pcom or if the Pcom can be controlled, such as when its origin is situated proximal to the aneurysm. If proximal control is not available, cervical ICA temporary occlusion or suction decompression via cervical exposure or an endovascular route must be used.

Clipping of anterior wall aneurysms can be accomplished by applying a large clip parallel to the direction of the ICA, with additional safety clips on top (Fig. 8.7). Multiple clips are often necessary because the closing force of the available clips is insufficient for a single clip to withstand the wall tension. As an alternative, a series of clips placed perpendicular to the carotid may be used. It is not always easy to appreciate the residual inner diameter of the reconstructed carotid exactly, so reconstruction should be aimed at achieving an artery that is a bit too wide rather than too narrow. Control of patency with micro-Doppler and ICG angiography is also important.

Back wall aneurysms can be clipped by passing straight or slightly curved clips beneath the ICA, though it may be difficult to align clip direction with the line of the ICA. Using a series of angled, fenestrated clips that embrace the ICA often may be a better alternative. When using this technique, the resulting vessel diameter will usually be smaller than anticipated. We recommend advancing the clip 1 mm deeper than is intuitively felt correct at first.

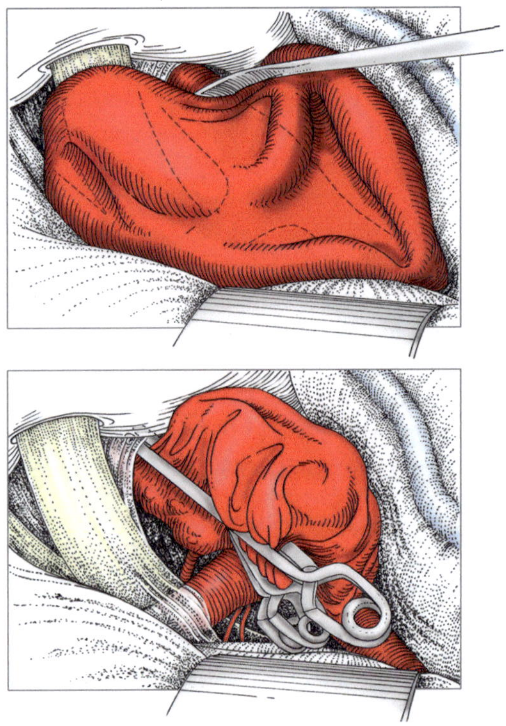

Fig. 8.7 Collapsed aneurysm after temporary clipping, suction decompression, or induced hypotension. Clip reconstruction with multiple clips

8.5 Aneurysms of the Internal Carotid Artery Bifurcation

8.5.1 General Considerations

ICA bifurcation aneurysms represent 2–8 % of all aneurysms. They are reported to be more frequent than other intracranial aneurysms in younger patients [10]. The main difficulty in microneurosurgical management of these aneurysms is preserving flow in all the perforators surrounding or adherent to the aneurysm dome.

ICA bifurcation aneurysms are well suited for the endovascular approach, and a decision favoring endovascular therapy should generally be made in the case of SAH unless the aneurysm appears difficult for endovascular treatment because of size or neck configuration. This shift of paradigm means that more complex cases are left for microsurgical treatment. The choice of treatment modality for unruptured aneurysms is a matter for discussion particularly in this location, because these aneurysms are more common in younger patients, for whom a permanent and stable solution is essential.

Preservation of flow in the perforating branches of the ICA bifurcation is the main challenge for microsurgical therapy. The concerned branches correspond to the proximal diencephalic perforators of the anterior and middle cerebral artery and Heubner's retrograde artery, which usually curves around the back side of the aneurysm neck. The functional consequences of perforator occlusion in this area, including infarction of Heubner's territory, are highly variable and are not amenable to electrophysiological monitoring. Nonetheless, the use of intraoperative monitoring is recommended, particularly with large or otherwise complex aneurysms, in order for the surgeon to be alerted about potential compromise of flow in the middle cerebral artery (MCA) and anterior cerebral artery (ACA) and to monitor tolerance of temporary clipping.

8.5.2 Dissection and Clipping

The anatomical projection of the fundus of ICA bifurcation aneurysms has not been well studied because of their relative rarity. There is little doubt, however, that they obey the general principles as outlined earlier. Most often, the aneurysms form an elongation of the afferent terminal ICA, with a slight tilt upward or downward, with the upward tilt being more common (Fig. 8.8).

A pterional craniotomy is chosen for these aneurysms. Positioning is the same as for the other ICA aneurysms. The Sylvian fissure must be completely opened, and it is necessary to use a retractor blade on the frontal and temporal lobes.

Gaining proximal control is usually not a problem with these aneurysms. The terminal ICA comes into sight first after splitting of the Sylvian fissure. The suprachiasmatic cisterns are opened sufficiently to enable mobilization of the posterior aspect of the orbital cortex, and the origins of the proximal segment of the MCA (M1) and the precommunicating segment of the ACA (A1) are dissected free.

The aneurysm neck then is prepared for clipping; small perforators are carefully dissected off the aneurysm neck. We feel that is important to use nimodipine irrigation, particularly when dissection of perforators is necessary.

The principal indication to use temporary clipping in this location is the same as for other sites. If complete trapping of the ICA bifurcation becomes necessary, however, the short ischemic tolerance of the affected perforators must be kept in mind. Long temporary occlusion times that may be well tolerated at the MCA bifurcation, for example, are not recommended.

The direction of clip application has a certain importance in this location. It is important to keep in mind the final position of the orbital cortex after removal of the retractor blade. The head of the clip must lie in the Sylvian fissure; otherwise, it may be twisted by the weight of the orbital cortex, resulting in compression of the A1 or M1 root.

Following clip application, the result must be very carefully inspected. The aneurysm must be collapsed in order to see the back side clearly. ICG angiography is very helpful to confirm the integrity of the perforators and identify obliteration. On the other hand, the value of micro-Doppler to confirm flow in the perforators must be seen critically. These arteries are too small to provide a good signal, and the special resolution of the available probe does not allow to distinguish between neighboring perforators with certainty.

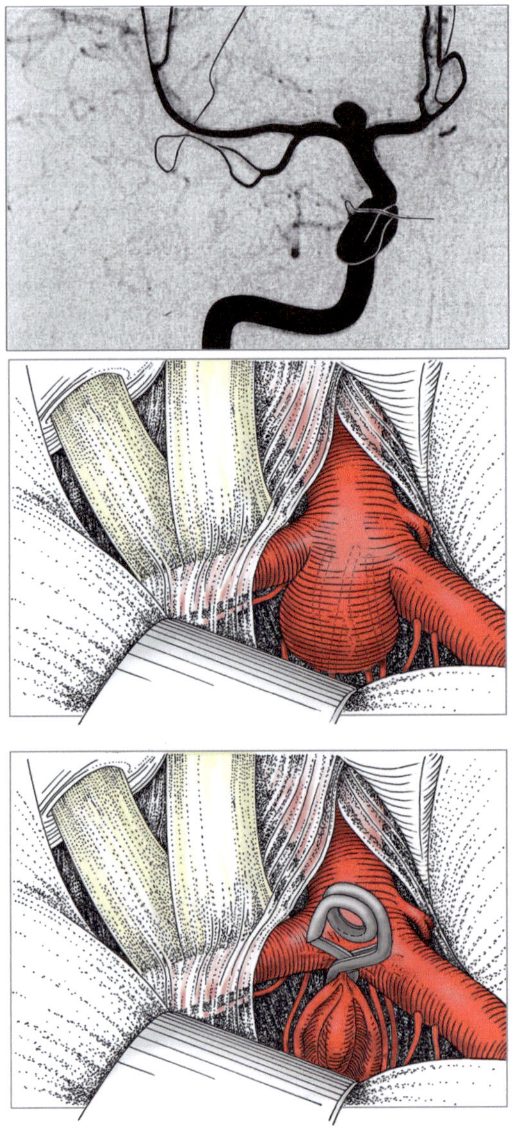

Fig. 8.8 Digital subtraction angiography showing ICA bifurcation aneurysm. Perforators must be carefully separated (operative view). Clip positioning

References

1. Batjer HH, Samson DS. Retrograde suction decompression of giant paraclinoidal aneurysms. Technical note. J Neurosurg. 1990;73:305–6.
2. Lam AM. The choice of controlled hypotension during repair of intracranial aneurysms: techniques and complications. Agressologie. 1990;31:357–9.
3. Guinn NR, McDonagh DL, Borel CO, Wright DR, Zomorodi AR, Powers CJ, et al. Adenosine-induced transient asystole for intracranial aneurysm surgery: a retrospective review. J Neurosurg Anesthesiol. 2011; 23:35–40.
4. Sanai N, Caldwell N, Englot DJ, Lawton MT. Advanced technical skills are required for microsurgical clipping of posterior communicating artery aneurysms in the endovascular era. Neurosurgery. 2012;71:285–94; discussion 294–5.
5. Cho MS, Kim MS, Chang CH, Kim SW, Kim SH, Choi BY. Analysis of clip-induced ischemic complication of anterior choroidal artery aneurysms. J Korean Neurosurg Soc. 2008;43:131–4.
6. Tanaka Y, Kobayashi S, Kyoshima K, Sugita K. Multiple clipping technique for large and giant internal carotid artery aneurysms and complications: angiographic analysis. J Neurosurg. 1994;80:635–42.
7. Sano H. Treatment of complex intracranial aneurysms of anterior circulation using multiple clips. Acta Neurochir Suppl. 2010;107:27–31.
8. Yasargil MG. Microneurosurgery, vol. 1. Stuttgart: Thieme; 1984. p. 260ff.
9. Hongo K, Horiuchi T, Nitta J, Tanaka Y, Tada T, Kobayashi S. Double-insurance bypass for internal carotid artery aneurysm surgery. Neurosurgery. 2003;52:597–602; discussion 600–2.
10. Mehrotra A, Nair AP, Das KK, Srivastava A, Sahu RN, Kumar R. Clinical and radiological profiles and outcomes in pediatric patients with intracranial aneurysms. J Neurosurg Pediatr. 2012;10:340–6.

Suggested Reading

Friedman JA, Pichelmann MA, Piepgras DG, Atkinson JL, Maher CO, Meyer FB, Hansen KK. Ischemic complications of surgery for anterior choroidal artery aneurysms. J Neurosurg. 2001;94:565–72.

Grand W. Microsurgical anatomy of the proximal middle cerebral artery and the internal carotid artery bifurcation. Neurosurgery. 1980;7:215–8.

Güresir E, Schuss P, Setzer M, Platz J, Seifert V, Vatter H. Posterior communicating artery aneurysm–related oculomotor nerve palsy: influence of surgical and endovascular treatment on recovery: single-center series and systematic review. Neurosurgery. 2011;68:1527–33; discussion 1533–4.

Heros RC, Nelson PB, Ojemann RG, Crowell RM, DeBrun G. Large and giant paraclinoid aneurysms: surgical techniques, complications, and results. Neurosurgery. 1983;12:153–63.

Hokama M, Hongo K, Gibo H, Kyoshima K, Kobayashi S. Microsurgical anatomy of the ophthalmic artery and the distal dural ring for the juxta-dural ring aneurysms via the pterional approach. Neurol Res. 2001;23:331–5.

Lehecka M, Dashti R, Romani R, Celik O, Navratil O, Kivipelto L, et al. Microneurosurgical management of internal carotid artery bifurcation aneurysms. Surg Neurol. 2009;71:649–67.

Pikus HJ, Heros RC. Surgical treatment of internal carotid and posterior communicating artery aneurysms. Neurosurg Clin N Am. 1998;9:785–95.

Scott JA, Horner TG, Leipzig TJ. Retrograde suction decompression of an ophthalmic artery aneurysm using balloon occlusion. Technical note. J Neurosurg. 1991;75:146–7.

Vincentelli F, Caruso G, Grisoli F, Rabehanta P, Andriamamonjy C, Gouaze A. Microsurgical anatomy of the cisternal course of the perforating branches of the posterior communicating artery. Neurosurgery. 1990;26:824–31.

9 Aneurysms of the Vertebral Artery and Branches

9.1 General Considerations

Aneurysms of the posterior cerebral circulation account for only about 15 % of all intracranial aneurysms, and surgical treatment of these aneurysms was demanding until the introduction of endovascular therapy. The surgery-related morbidity and mortality—about 10 % in the best published series—was correspondingly high. One must assume that in the average series, the surgery-related morbidity and mortality may have been about 30 % or higher. Part of the high complication rate can be linked to the relative rarity of these aneurysms, because the particular approaches and techniques require special skills and awareness of specific pitfalls. Another reason for the unsatisfactory results of microsurgical treatment, however, has certainly been the highly eloquent territory supplied by the parent arteries of these aneurysms—that is, the brainstem. Drake and Peerless from London, Ontario, acquired the world's largest experience in the surgical treatment of aneurysms of the posterior circulation [1].

The difficult surgical therapy for aneurysms of the basilar artery led to the acceptance of endovascular therapy as the treatment of first choice prior to the general acceptance of endovascular coiling. In the late 1990s, it was shown that the treatment-related morbidity and mortality after endovascular treatment was lower than after microsurgical operation. Thus, the endovascular treatment of basilar artery aneurysms was established 3–4 years before the general acceptance of endovascular therapy for ruptured aneurysms in the wake of the International Subarachnoid Aneurysm Trial (ISAT), the results of which were first published in 2002.

The acceptance of the superiority of endovascular treatment techniques applies not to all aneurysms in the posterior circulation, but particularly to aneurysms of the basilar artery. Of all ruptured and unruptured aneurysms of the posterior circulation, the aneurysms of the basilar bifurcation account for approximately 50 %. The next most common locations are the origin of the superior cerebellar artery (SCA) and the origin of the posterior inferior cerebellar artery (PICA), each with about 15 %. Other sites of saccular and fusiform aneurysms of the posterior circulation are the junction of the vertebral arteries and the origin of the anterior inferior cerebellar artery (AICA). Aneurysms occur rarely at the origin of the posterior communicating artery from the posterior cerebral artery, as well as in the peripheral portions of the posterior cerebral artery and the peripheral portions of the SCA, AICA, and PICA. These latter groups each account for a few percent of all aneurysms of the posterior circulation. Special situations are dissecting aneurysms, especially of the vertebral artery, fusiform vertebrobasilar aneurysms in the context of arterial ectasia and elongation (megadolichobasilar artery), and aneurysms of the feeder arteries of posterior fossa arteriovenous malformations. Each of these special situations accounts also for a few of all aneurysms of the posterior circulation.

H.-J. Steiger et al., *Microsurgical Brain Aneurysms: Illustrated Concepts and Cases*,
DOI 10.1007/978-3-662-45679-8_9, © Springer-Verlag Berlin Heidelberg 2015

Endovascular treatment of aneurysms of the basilar bifurcation and aneurysms at the origin of the SCA and AICA has become so well established that microsurgical competence has been lost and microsurgical therapy is no longer available as an alternative for these aneurysms. The situation for saccular aneurysms at the origin of the PICA from the vertebral artery is different; both endovascular and microsurgical therapies currently appear to be equivalent [2]. It remains unclear which treatment modality provides better short-term and long-term results, on the average. Finally, endovascular treatment of peripheral aneurysms is currently difficult. From the endovascular side, only obliteration of the carrier artery may be offered, which generally results in territorial cerebellar infarction. Therefore, peripheral aneurysms remain the domain of microsurgery.

9.1.1 PICA Aneurysms

The PICA is characterized by a highly variable origin: In 90 % of individuals, it originates from the so-called intradural V4 segment of the vertebral artery, and in about 10 % it originates extracranially from the extradural V3 segment of the vertebral artery, or from the basilar artery. Anatomically, the PICA runs in a tortuous way around the lateral medulla oblongata at the level of the caudal cranial nerves (IX–XII). At the anterior aspect of the cerebellar tonsil, it forms the caudal loop. In its further course, the PICA runs between the dorsal aspect of the medulla oblongata and the tonsils and forms the cranial loop. The distal portion divides into two main branches to supply the vermis and cerebellar hemisphere [3].

In principle, the PICA is divided into five sections: (1) anteromedullary, (2) lateromedullary, (3) tonsillomedullary, (4) telovelotonsillary, and (5) the cortical segment. The rami perforantes arise from the first three segments to supply the posterolateral medulla. The first three segments are also referred to as the proximal PICA; segments four and five are the distal PICA. About 2 % of all intracranial aneurysms are associated with the PICA. Clinically, PICA aneurysms may present with rupture and consecutive subarachnoid hemorrhage (SAH), or conversely with signs of ischemia or as an expression of a mass, with symptoms such as hiccups, dysphagia, and other paralytic caudal cranial nerve failures.

PICA-origin aneurysms are most common. As mentioned, both endovascular and surgical treatment modalities are currently used for optimal care. Details of the surgical management are given in a subsequent section.

9.1.2 AICA Aneurysms

The AICA originates anatomically from the lower third of the basilar artery, in the prepontine region of the cerebellopontine angle. It is surrounded by numerous caudal cranial nerves and the arterial perforators of the brain stem. Less than 1 % of all intracranial aneurysms may be associated with the AICA. Most AICA aneurysms become symptomatic with SAH, but giant aneurysms (>2.5 cm) represent a significant proportion and become symptomatic by signs of brainstem compression.

Aneurysms with AICA origin are difficult to access surgically, which is the main reason that endovascular therapy has been accepted as the first treatment choice.

9.1.3 Dissecting Aneurysms of the Vertebral Artery

Anatomically, the vertebral artery runs anteriorly from the transverse foramen of the atlas, ascending dorsally and medially to the atlanto-occipital joint and entering the subarachnoid space at the level of the occipital condyle. Intracranial dissecting aneurysms occur preferentially at the proximal intradural vertebral artery. Mechanical stress is considered to be a pathophysiological factor. Dissecting aneurysms occur more frequently in the vertebrobasilar territory than in the carotid artery.

Dissecting aneurysms can result in ischemia by vascular occlusion or thromboembolism, compression of surrounding structures, or rupture with SAH. Because of the generally good collateral circulation of the brainstem, with inflows of both vertebral arteries and connections to the carotid artery by the posterior communicating arteries, dissection of a vertebral artery leads only in exceptional cases to direct hemodynamic compromise, but thromboembolic complications can lead to basilar thrombosis or embolic occlusion of the posterior cerebral arteries.

Thromboembolic complications today can be effectively prevented pharmacologically, and the prognosis of dissecting aneurysms with nonhemorrhagic manifestation appears relatively good. The prognosis for ruptured dissecting aneurysms with SAH, on the other hand, must be regarded as highly critical; the rate of rerupture is higher than with saccular aneurysms.

The typical angiographic feature of a dissecting aneurysm is the "pearl and string" sign—a dilated arterial segment next to a narrowed segment—but sometimes only discrete changes of arterial caliber are evident. These changes often are detectable only with catheter angiography, as the resolution of CT angiography or MR angiography is not sufficient to detect such small changes in caliber. Definition of intramural hematoma on MRI is the key finding for diagnosis of an extradural arterial dissection, but attempts to use this feature to identify intradural dissections have been disappointing, particularly in the context of SAH.

Dissecting vertebral artery aneurysms can be treated by an endovascular route or microsurgically. With both options, the main questions during planning are whether arterial continuity must be preserved and whether it can be preserved. Preservation of the vascular continuity is possible via the endovascular route with the help of stents or flow diverters [4]. Microsurgically, preservation of the arterial continuity is possible with the help of encircling clips or wrapping [5].

The original publications in the past 10 years regarding treatment of intracranial dissecting vertebral artery aneurysms show a clear trend toward endovascular therapy. It appears that surgical therapy has largely been abandoned in favor of endovascular treatment. There is also an evident trend away from the occlusion of the parent artery toward continuity-conserving therapy using stents.

The primary objective is to prevent the rerupture of the dissecting aneurysm. The easiest way to prevent rerupture is occlusion of the parent artery. Often, the branches of the dissected vessel segment are already occluded by the dissection, so that locally branching arteries are less relevant in weighing the pros and cons of vessel occlusion. More important is the appreciation of the hemodynamic importance of the affected artery. The hemodynamic significance extends from "not relevant" in the case of a hypoplastic vessel or well-collateralized artery to "hemodynamically essential," describing a vessel that cannot be sacrificed. In these latter situations, it is necessary to preserve continuity by means of endovascular stents or flow diverters. Flow diverters carry a risk of occluding perforators and branches originating from the arterial segments immediately adjacent to the dissection, where the device must be anchored. The inflows to the anterior spinal artery, the PICA, and the branches to the dorsolateral medulla oblongata especially must be taken into consideration in the intradural portions of the vertebral artery.

9.1.4 Dolichoectatic Vertebrobasilar Aneurysms

Dolichoectatic widening of the basilar artery is usually associated with long-standing hypertension and generalized arteriosclerosis. Accordingly, it mainly affects patients in the sixth and seventh decades of life. Symptoms result from slow and progressive brainstem compression, ischemia by thrombosis and perforator occlusion, and SAH.

Treatment of these aneurysms, whether endovascular or microsurgical, is problematic. Anson and colleagues [6] published their surgical experience in the 1990s, reporting reasonable results in view of the complexity of the aneurysms and the comorbidity of the patients. Nonetheless, reports in recent years signal a clear shift toward endovascular therapy. In the light of the generally high treatment risk, invasive treatment should be restricted to ruptured aneurysms with SAH. Unruptured cases presenting ischemic symptoms should be treated with platelet aggregation inhibitors. Treatment decisions about aneurysms presenting with mass effect are particularly difficult. At the moment, it remains questionable whether interventional treatment provides any benefit.

In patients presenting with SAH, a decision favoring active treatment appears relatively straightforward despite the actual lack of data regarding risk and benefit, but we recommend limiting intervention to the minimum necessary to prevent rerupture. It is sometimes possible to locate the point of rupture (e.g., a saccular formation). We recommend protecting only this area with the help of stent-assisted endovascular coiling.

9.1.5 Feeder Aneurysms with Cerebellar Arteriovenous Malformation

Hemorrhage in an arteriovenous malformation (AVM) of the cerebellum may arise from saccular aneurysms of the feeding vessels. These aneurysms are formally peripheral SCA, AICA, or PICA aneurysms. Here the posterior circulation differs somewhat from the supratentorial situation, in which aneurysms on the feeding vessels (though well known) appear to be much less frequently the cause of bleeding. This specific feature of AVMs of the posterior fossa was first worked out by Westphal and Grzyska [7]. In contrast to other peripheral aneurysms of the cerebellar arteries, AVM-related aneurysms may be treated by endovascular or surgical occlusion of the parent artery.

9.2 Microsurgery of PICA Aneurysms

9.2.1 Vertebral Artery PICA-Origin Aneurysms

In principle, most PICA-origin aneurysms can be treated by the endovascular or microsurgical route. To date, it is unclear which method is superior. The small, monocentric series published do not allow comparison of the treatment results. Many PICA-origin aneurysms are relatively broad based and therefore particularly complicated for endovascular therapy. The main problem with the microsurgical approach is the nearness to the caudal cranial nerves, with the risk of damage.

For PICA-origin aneurysms, the most important factors in the initial interdisciplinary decision making with regard to treatment modality are (1) the level of PICA origin in relation to the vertebral artery and the brainstem and (2) the shape of the aneurysm. High-lying prepontine aneurysm locations are difficult to approach microsurgically, and in these situations, the endovascular approach appears more favorable. On the other hand, a broad-based aneurysm—particularly if the PICA arises from the aneurysm—is difficult for endovascular therapy and should rather be approached microsurgically. During the planning phase, three-dimensional CT or MRI angiography reconstructions are helpful (Fig. 9.1).

Because of the proximity to the caudal cranial nerves, electrophysiological monitoring (i.e., somatosensory and motor-evoked potentials and electromyography of cranial nerves IX to XII) is useful and should be requested if possible.

We recommend the so-called park bench position for surgery on patients with PICA aneurysms. Access to proximal PICA aneurysms is gained via a lateral suboccipital craniectomy, with the inclusion of the foramen magnum (*see* Fig. 9.1). A far lateral approach is not necessary if the aneurysm is located lateral to the brainstem. A far lateral approach may be helpful for high-lying PICA origins and aneurysms lying in front of the brainstem, close to the vertebral junction [8]. It is important to maintain the functional portion of the occipital condyles. For low-lying aneurysms, it may rarely be necessary to extend the craniectomy caudally via a hemilaminectomy of the arch of C1.

After arc-shaped opening of the dura mater and the cisterna magna, the ipsilateral cerebellar tonsil is slightly elevated. The vertebral artery is then identified medial and rostral to the dentate ligament; the origin of the PICA is usually seen between the fascicles of the caudal cranial nerves (Fig. 9.2). More distally located PICA origins are in contact with the fascicles of the glossopharyngeal and vagus nerves, and more proximal origins are in contact with the fascicles of the accessory and hypoglossal nerves [3, 9]. Fenestrated or slightly curved aneurysm clips can be useful in order to avoid injury to these fascicles.

Following clip application and verification of complete occlusion and patency of the PICA by micro-Doppler and indocyanine green (ICG) video angiography, it is important to pay attention to watertight closure of the dura. Dural leaks are a particularly annoying complication that results in space-occupying pseudomeningocele, possibly followed by hydrocephalus or even cervical syringomyelia.

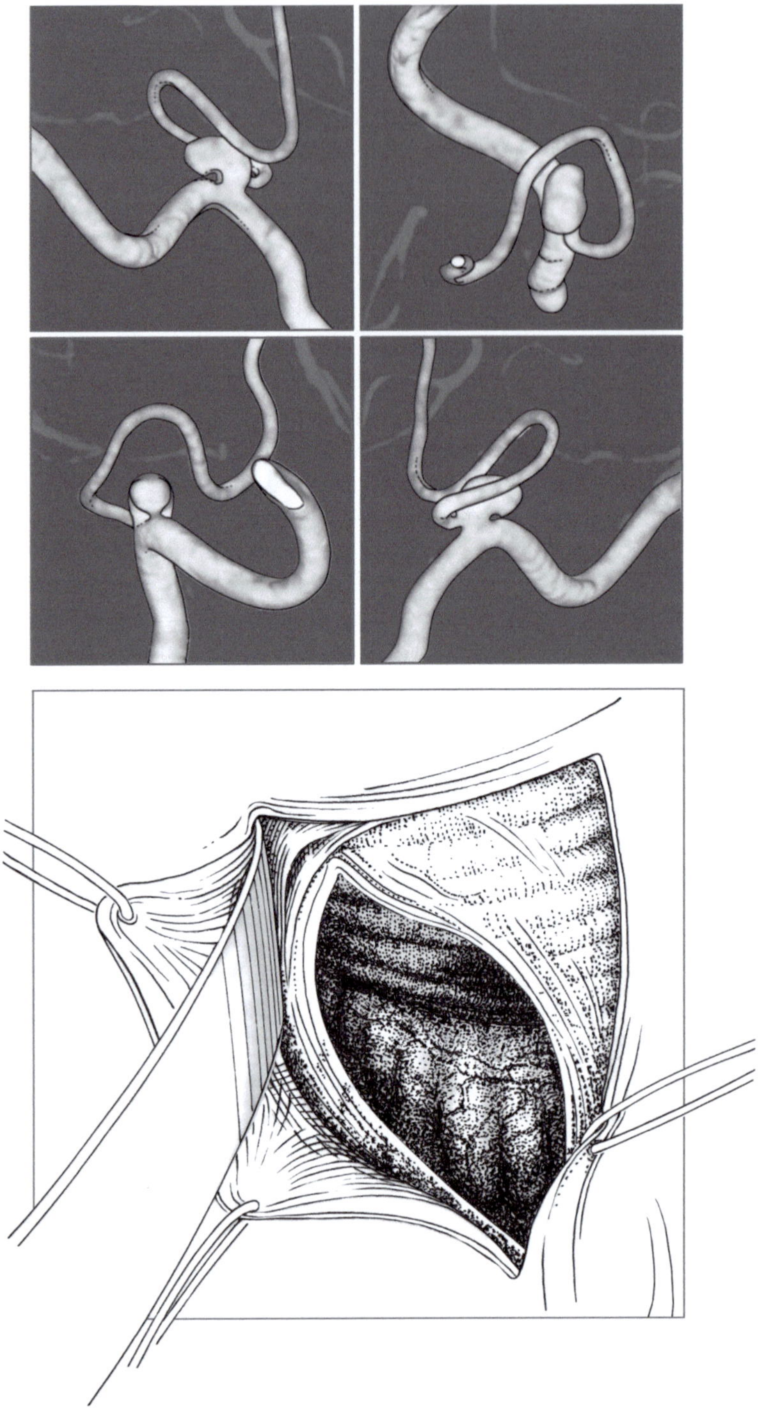

Fig. 9.1 Three-dimensional angiographic images of a ruptured right-sided vertebral artery aneurysm at the bifurcation of the posterior inferior cerebral artery (PICA). Slightly lateralized, right-sided suboccipital midline craniotomy

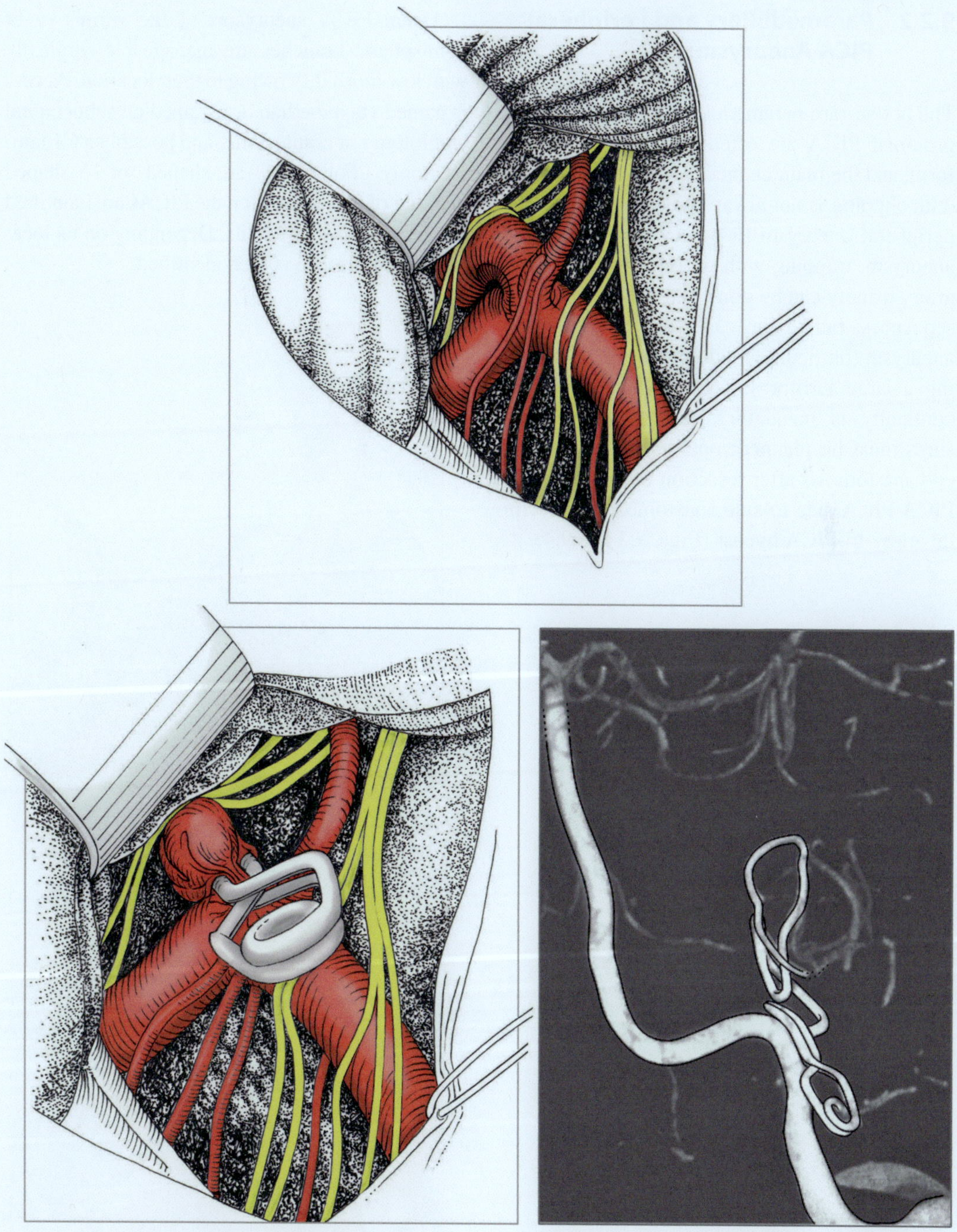

Fig. 9.2 Mild retraction of the right cerebellar tonsils and cerebellum to approach the vertebral artery and the PICA aneurysm. Following careful dissection of the lower cranial nerves, the aneurysm is clipped with a curved aneurysm clip. Postoperative catheter angiography

9.2.2 Paramedullary and Peripheral PICA Aneurysms

The not-so-rare paramedullary aneurysms on the proximal PICA are often broad based or fusiform, and the maintenance of vascular continuity with clipping is not always possible. In case of a peripheral aneurysm or an AVM-related feeder aneurysm, trapping with occlusion of the parent artery usually can be done without negative consequences, but in the case of a paramedullary aneurysm (particularly a dominant PICA supplying a large territory), preservation of vascular continuity is mandatory. Reconstructive measures must be planned; options include end-to-end anastomosis after resection of the aneurysm, PICA-PICA side-to-side anastomosis, or occipital artery-to-PICA bypass (Figs. 9.3 and 9.4).

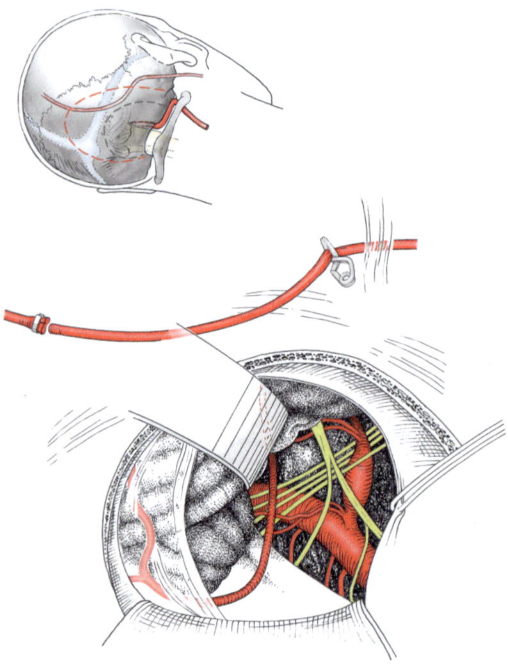

Fig. 9.3 Schematic illustration of the occipital artery (OA) and the dominant vertebral artery, the skin incision (*dashed red line*), and craniotomy (*dashed black line*) for planned paramedullary aneurysm trapping and revascularization of the distal PICA by an occipital artery-to-PICA bypass. Following dissection of the OA, the dissecting aneurysm of the PICA is approached

Distal PICA aneurysms of the vermis or of hemispheric branches are manageable surgically with low morbidity owing to their location. Access is gained via a median or paramedian suboccipital craniotomy or craniectomy and possibly a C1 laminectomy. Following arc-shaped or Y-shaped opening of the dura mater, the PICAs are identified between cerebellar tonsils. Depending on its location, the aneurysm is then identified.

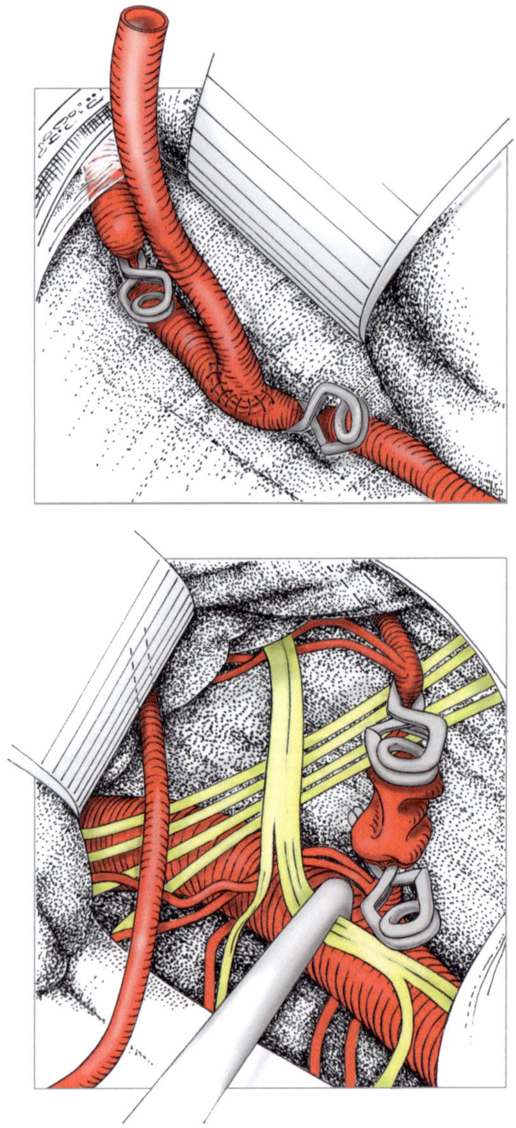

Fig. 9.4 An OA-PICA bypass is performed in the distal (fifth) tonsillar segment of the PICA. The dissecting aneurysm is trapped, preferably distal to the PICA perforating arteries

References

1. Drake CG, Peerless SJ, Hernesniemi JA. Surgery of vertebrobasilar aneurysms: London, Ontario, experience on 1,767 patients. New York: Springer; 1996.
2. Lehto H, Harati A, Niemelä M, Dashti R, Laakso A, Elsharkawy A, et al. Distal posterior inferior cerebellar artery aneurysms: clinical features and outcome of 80 patients. World Neurosurg. 2014. doi:10.1016/j.wneu.2014.06.012.
3. Rodriguez-Hernandez A, Rhoton Jr AL, Lawton MT. Segmental anatomy of the cerebellar arteries: a proposed nomenclature. Laboratory investigation. J Neurosurg. 2011;115:387–97.
4. Park SI, Kim BM, Kim DI, Shin YS, Suh SH, Chung EC, et al. Clinical and angiographic follow-up of stent-only therapy for acute intracranial vertebrobasilar dissecting aneurysms. AJNR Am J Neuroradiol. 2009;30:1351–6.
5. Uhl E, Schmid-Elsaesser R, Steiger HJ. Ruptured intracranial dissecting aneurysms: management considerations with a focus on surgical and endovascular techniques to preserve arterial continuity. Acta Neurochir (Wien). 2003;145:1073–83; discussion 1083–4.
6. Anson JA, Lawton MT, Spetzler RF. Characteristics and surgical treatment of dolichoectatic and fusiform aneurysms. J Neurosurg. 1996;84:185–93.
7. Westphal M, Grzyska U. Clinical significance of pedicle aneurysms on feeding vessels, especially those located in infratentorial arteriovenous malformations. J Neurosurg. 2000;92:995–1001.
8. D'Ambrosio AL, Kreiter KT, Bush CA, Sciacca RR, Mayer SA, Solomon RA, Connolly Jr ES. Far lateral suboccipital approach for the treatment of proximal posteroinferior cerebellar artery aneurysms: surgical results and long-term outcome. Neurosurgery. 2004; 55:39–50.
9. Al-Khayat H, Al-Khayat H, Beshay J, Manner D, White J. Vertebral artery-posteroinferior cerebellar artery aneurysms: clinical and lower cranial nerve outcomes in 52 patients. Neurosurgery. 2005;56:2–10; discussion 11.

10 Some Complex Aneurysms and Solutions

10.1 General Considerations

Complex solutions for large, fusiform, and otherwise atypical aneurysms have been favorite topics of publications regarding technical aspects of aneurysm surgery over the past three decades. It is important to consider and communicate expectations and risks clearly before considering a nonstandard approach for a difficult constellation. By definition, the individual types of complex aneurysms are rare, so specific questions are hardly amenable to a formal study. Therefore, the options are most often considered and discussed only when the physician is confronted with a concrete situation. In general, nonstandardized surgical procedures belong to the category of "individualized treatment of a patient without scientifically proven benefit." Such procedures are acceptable if no other therapy is available.

Very often, some case reports are available when deciding upon an individualized treatment modality. Unfortunately, these reports of cases or small series do not help to assess risks and expectations, as these reports are particularly unbalanced on account of a large publication bias: Usually only cases with a positive outcome are published. Furthermore, we must be aware of the importance of the logical consistency of the treatment concept—or the lack of it. If the planned procedure can be subdivided into a series of standard steps with known success rates and risks, the risk of the complete operation can be more concretely grasped than if this is not possible. Nonetheless, in this situation, there is some interconnection between known standard procedures that may result in uncertainty. For example, let us consider that we plan to use a balloon-assisted technique for remodeling and clip application, a technique that is well established for endovascular coiling of aneurysms. If the method is used during open surgery in a hybrid surgical-endovascular environment, however, the balloon probably will have to stay in place longer, and the possibilities of anticoagulation and thrombolysis are more limited, resulting in an increased risk compared with the purely endovascular setting. Furthermore, the interaction between clip and balloon may differ from the interaction between coil and balloon. The clip might tack the balloon, preventing retrieval, leading to rupture of the balloon, and so forth.

It appears reasonable to assume that neither existing reports on a special technique nor an apparently sound logical concept provides a guarantee that the concept will work in practice. For the situation of a complex aneurysm, it therefore appears reasonable to assume a 50 % chance that a new treatment concept will work. If after an initial successful outcome, the same concept is applied for subsequent cases, the chance of success increases. After some ten cases, a gross assessment of the chances of success and the risks can be made. If such a series is planned, however, consent of the institutional ethics committee is now required.

H.-J. Steiger et al., *Microsurgical Brain Aneurysms: Illustrated Concepts and Cases*,
DOI 10.1007/978-3-662-45679-8_10, © Springer-Verlag Berlin Heidelberg 2015

10.2 Paraclinoid Giant Aneurysm: Balloon-Assisted Clipping

Large and giant proximal internal carotid artery (ICA) aneurysms present a therapeutic challenge. These aneurysms frequently require the temporary interruption of local circulation to facilitate safe occlusion. Owing to the brisk retrograde blood flow through the ophthalmic artery and cavernous branches, simple trapping of the aneurysm by cervical ICA clamping and intracranial distal clipping may not adequately soften the aneurysm. Retrograde aspiration via a catheter inserted in the cervical ICA was introduced by Batjer and Samson [1] (see also Chap. 8). We introduced balloon-assisted temporary blockage of aneurysmal flow and decompression by blocking the entire orifice of the aneurysm with a longitudinal intracarotid balloon [2].

In this procedure, a latex balloon 15–20 mm long is advanced into the carotid siphon so that the markers of the proximal and distal end of the balloon are visible proximal and distal to the aneurysmal neck. Following dissection of the aneurysm, the inserted balloon is inflated under angiographic control until the ICA is completely blocked (Fig. 10.1). After confirmation that the neck is soft and pliable, the aneurysm is clipped by several large clips. The balloon is subsequently deflated and removed.

In the few cases in which this method has been applied, major thromboembolic complications did not occur, and the aneurysms could be clipped well. In one case of an unruptured aneurysm, however, transient pronounced vasospasm occurred postoperatively. The causal relation to the use of the balloon remains unclear [2].

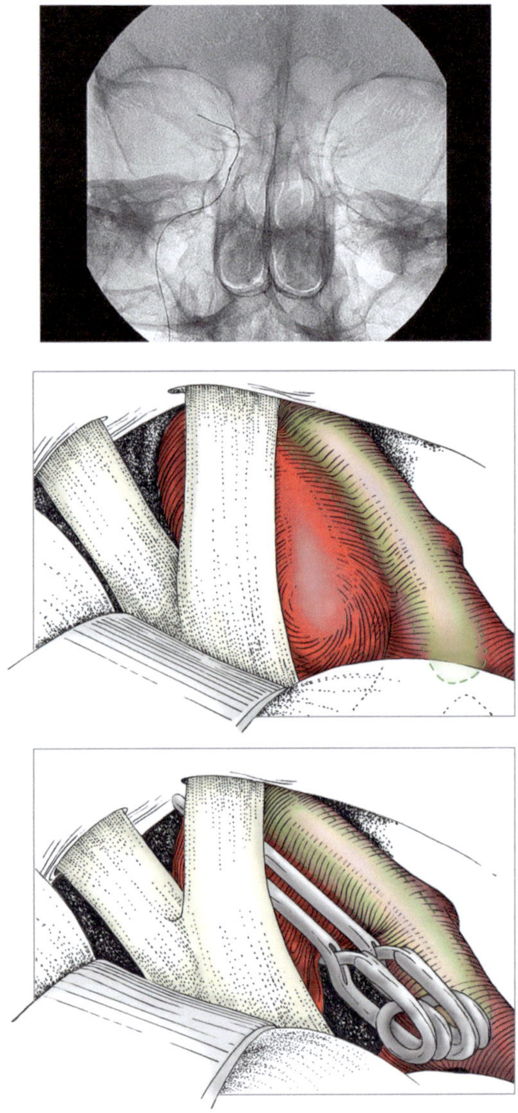

Fig. 10.1 Balloon-assisted clipping of a giant paraclinoid aneurysm. The balloon catheter is advanced into the carotid siphon until the markers of the proximal and distal end of the balloon cover the assumed neck of the aneurysm. Following dissection of the aneurysm, the balloon is inflated to occlude the internal carotid artery and the blood flow into the aneurysm. After confirming by palpation with the dissector that the aneurysm has become soft and pliable, it can be clipped with several large clips

10.3 Fusiform Aneurysm: Bypass and Coil Occlusion

Fusiform aneurysms are not amenable to clipping and need to be treated by elimination of the concerned vascular segment. In general, the distal vascular territories need to be revascularized unless balloon test occlusion proves that there is sufficient collateral flow [3]. A further concern is the perforators potentially originating from the fusiform aneurysm. In cases of circumferential thrombosis within the aneurysm, it can be assumed that there are no functional perforators. The choice of bypass methods remains a matter of discussion. Standard extracranial to intracranial (EC-IC) bypass using the superficial temporal artery achieves a limited amount of flow. The methods of assessment of the flow demand and the flow potential of a donor artery have been conceptually defined by Amin-Hanjani and colleagues [4–6]. Standard EC-IC bypasses are a time-proven method with high long-term patency rates (Figs. 10.2 and 10.3). If the flow demand is higher than the potential supply by the available superficial temporal artery, a high-flow bypass using a vein or radial artery graft must be used. These interposition bypasses carry a higher periprocedural risk, however, along with lower long-term patency rates.

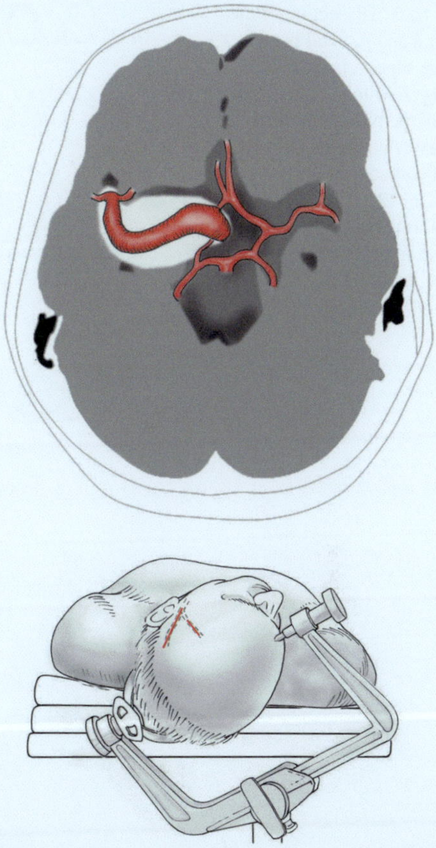

Fig. 10.2 Example of a fusiform, partially thrombosed aneurysm of the left proximal segment of the middle cerebral artery (M1 segment). Positioning for a planned double-barrel bypass using both branches of the superficial temporal artery

Fig. 10.3 Dissection of the frontal and parietal branches of the superficial temporal artery. End-to-side anastomoses of the two branches to an infrasylvian and a suprasylvian cortical artery, respectively. The entire fusiform aneurysm was subsequently filled with coils, resulting in complete thrombosis of the aneurysm

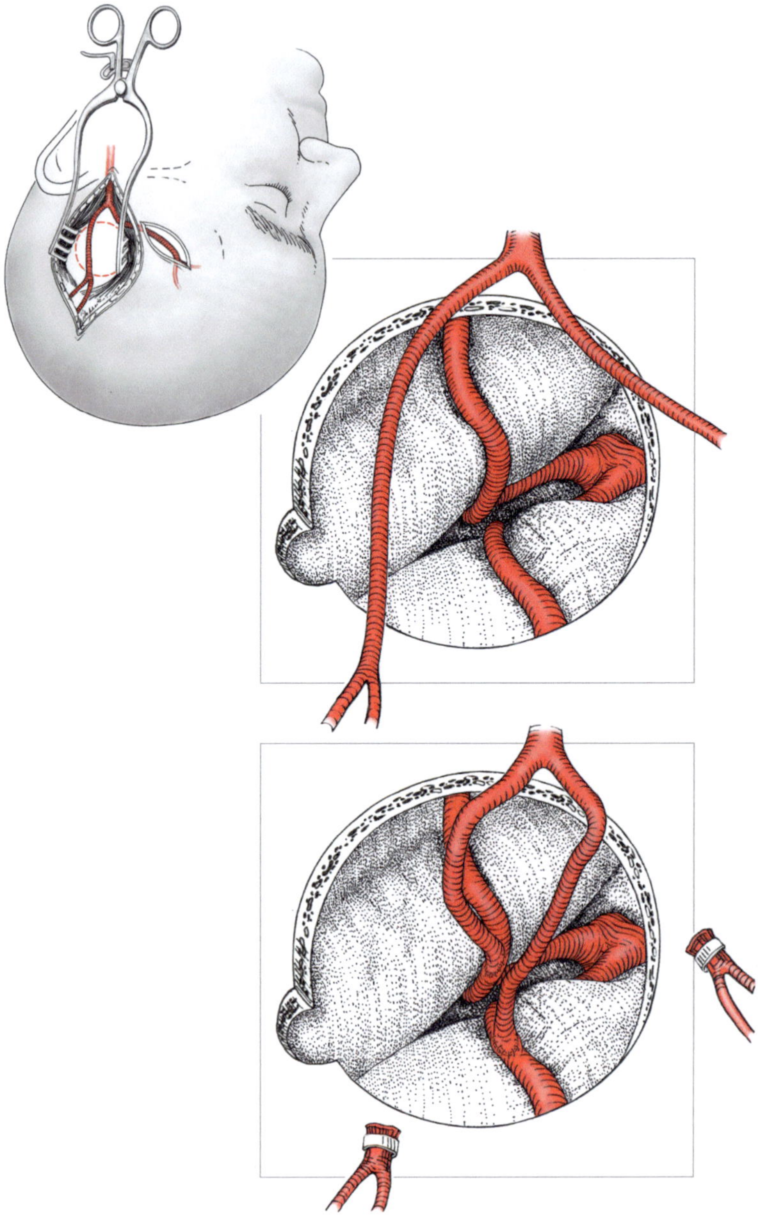

References

1. Batjer HH, Samson DS. Retrograde suction decompression of giant paraclinoidal aneurysms. Technical note. J Neurosurg. 1990;73:305–6.
2. Steiger HJ, Lins F, Mayer T, Schmid-Elsaesser R, Stummer W, Turowski B. Temporary aneurysm orifice balloon occlusion as an alternative to retrograde suction decompression for giant paraclinoid internal carotid artery aneurysms: technical note. Neurosurgery. 2005;56:E442.
3. Chen L, Kato Y, Sano H, Watanabe S, Yoneda M, Hayakawa M, et al. Management of complex, surgically intractable intracranial aneurysms: the option for intentional reconstruction of aneurysm neck followed by endovascular coiling. Cerebrovasc Dis. 2007;23:381–7.
4. Amin-Hanjani S, Chen PR, Chang SW, Spetzler RF. Long-term follow-up of giant serpentine MCA aneurysm treated with EC-IC bypass and proximal occlusion. Acta Neurochir (Wien). 2006;148: 227–8.
5. Amin-Hanjani S, Meglio G, Gatto R, Bauer A, Charbel FT. The utility of intraoperative blood flow measurement during aneurysm surgery using an ultrasonic perivascular flow probe. Neurosurgery. 2008; 62:1346–53.
6. Amin-Hanjani S, Alaraj A, Charbel FT. Flow replacement bypass for aneurysms: decision-making using intraoperative blood flow measurements. Acta Neurochir (Wien). 2010;152:1021–32; discussion 1032.

Peripheral and Mycotic Aneurysms 11

Peripheral aneurysms fall into three main categories:

- Saccular aneurysms located at bifurcations of the postcommunicating artery segments of the anterior or posterior cerebral artery or at bifurcations of the M2 and peripheral segments of the middle cerebral artery
- Mycotic or infectious aneurysms
- Aneurysms associated with arteriovenous malformations (AVMs)

All distal aneurysms are rare, and knowledge is based on reports of small case series. In addition to these main categories, cases of distal perforator aneurysms, peripheral dissecting aneurysms, and peripheral aneurysms in context with moyamoya disease also have been reported.

Peripheral aneurysms are therefore etiologically a mixed bag. Nonetheless, they share common features of clinical manifestations and therapeutic problems. They often present with intracerebral hemorrhage, sometimes in combination with cerebral infarction. They often have a relatively broad and thick-walled neck, which renders preservation of arterial continuity difficult during surgical or endovascular therapy. The aneurysm commonly needs to be trapped or the parent artery, occluded by the endovascular route, hoping for sufficient collateral flow to the concerned vascular territory. A further common denominator of the peripheral aneurysms is their variable location, calling for individual approaches. Image-guided navigation is mandatory for most peripheral aneurysms.

11.1 Saccular Aneurysms Located at Distal Bifurcations

11.1.1 General Considerations

Aneurysms located at distal bifurcations of the anterior, middle, or posterior cerebral arteries or cerebellar arteries are rare. Together, they appear to account for about 1 % of all aneurysms [1]. Several authors have pointed out that the incidence of multiple aneurysms is substantially higher in patients with distal aneurysms than has been reported in patients with proximal aneurysms, in whom multiplicity is seen in some 20 %. It remains unclear, therefore, whether some of these aneurysms have an infectious embolic origin—i.e., whether some should be classified instead as mycotic aneurysms.

Most often, distal bifurcation aneurysms are relatively small. They present with subarachnoid hemorrhage or intracerebral hematoma or rarely with acute subdural hematoma.

11.1.2 Approach and Clipping

Peripheral aneurysms of the anterior and posterior cerebral arteries lie within the interhemispheric fissure, and those arising from the middle cerebral artery are situated in the Sylvian fissure. Bifurcation-related peripheral aneurysms are rarely encountered on the brain surface. Functioning CSF drainage is important for all

H.-J. Steiger et al., *Microsurgical Brain Aneurysms: Illustrated Concepts and Cases*,
DOI 10.1007/978-3-662-45679-8_11, © Springer-Verlag Berlin Heidelberg 2015

procedures involving distal aneurysms located deeply in the interhemispheric or Sylvian fissure, as the surgical approach does not allow early access to CSF spaces to ensure sufficient brain relaxation.

Distal aneurysms of the anterior cerebral arteries are approached via an interhemispheric route, with the patient in a supine position. Distal aneurysms of the posterior cerebral arteries are usually approached via a posterior interhemispheric approach, with the patient in park bench position (Fig. 11.1). Exceptions are aneurysms of the postcommunicating segment of the posterior cerebral artery, which cannot be approached reasonably via the interhemispheric route. We believe that these aneurysms should be approached by an endovascular route whenever possible.

As mentioned above, the introduction of image-guided navigation has proven particularly useful for these distal aneurysms because of their variable location and the lack of reliable waypoints along the access route.

Although distal aneurysms are often quite small, measuring between 4 and 8 mm, their relation to the parent arteries is not very favorable. Particular care is required to preserve parent artery patency.

Fig. 11.1 Angiographic image of an unruptured distal posterior cerebral artery aneurysm, which became symptomatic with headache and visual auras. Left posterior interhemispheric parafalcine exposure and clipping

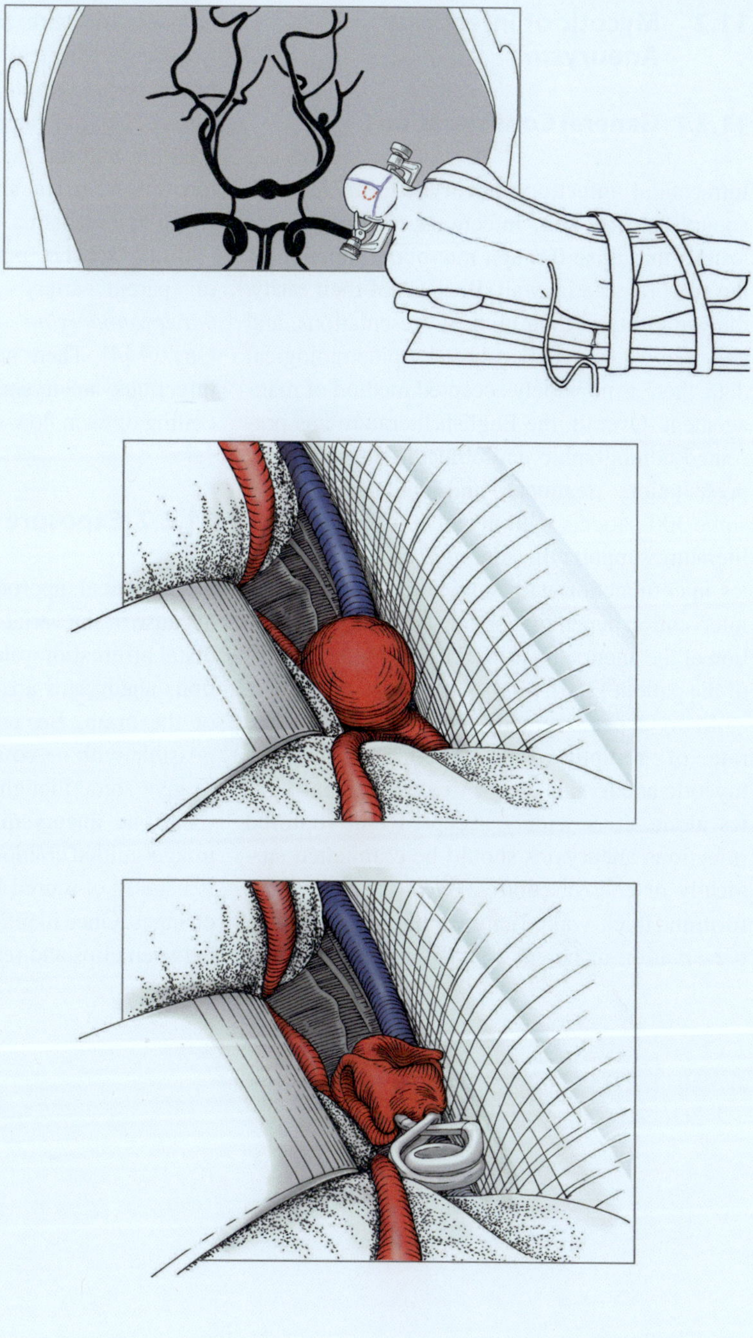

11.2 Mycotic or Infectious Aneurysms

11.2.1 General Considerations

Intracranial infectious aneurysms, or mycotic aneurysms, are rare, infectious cerebrovascular lesions that arise through microbial infection of the cerebral arterial wall. Because of their rarity, the variability in their clinical presentations, and the lack of population-based epidemiological data, there is no widely accepted method of management. Overall, the English literature has presented demographic and clinical data regarding presentation, treatment, and outcome of only some 300 patients with mycotic aneurysms. The literature supports the administration of antibiotics in conjunction with surgical or endovascular intervention depending on the character and location of the aneurysm, as well as the clinical status of the patient [2, 3].

Many aspects remain unclear, including the rate of rerupture and whether unruptured mycotic aneurysms can be treated with antibiotics alone. It is widely accepted that ruptured infectious aneurysms should be eliminated surgically or endovascularly. Because of the fusiform and thick-walled nature of these aneurysms, preservation of parent artery patency is usually not possible with either open or endovascular treatment. Surgical management usually comprises trapping and resection. A bypass procedure is not indicated because of the peripheral location and the fact that the supplied vascular territory is often already damaged by hemorrhage and ischemia.

Endovascular management usually consists of parent artery occlusion with coils, *n-butylcyanoacrylate*, ethylene vinyl alcohol, or Onyx® [4]. There are a few reports of proximal infectious aneurysms treated with direct stent-coiling or even flow-diverting stent monotherapy.

11.2.2 Exposure and Occlusion

The surgical approach must be individualized because of the variable location. In contrast to the distal bifurcation-related aneurysms, many infectious aneurysms are located close to the surface of the brain. Because flow preservation is not possible with mycotic aneurysms, it is important to give some thought to the vascular territory at risk. The aneurysm is exposed via a tailored image-guided craniotomy. The aneurysm contour is usually obscured by hemorrhage and reactive changes. Once identified, the aneurysm is trapped between clips and resected (Fig. 11.2).

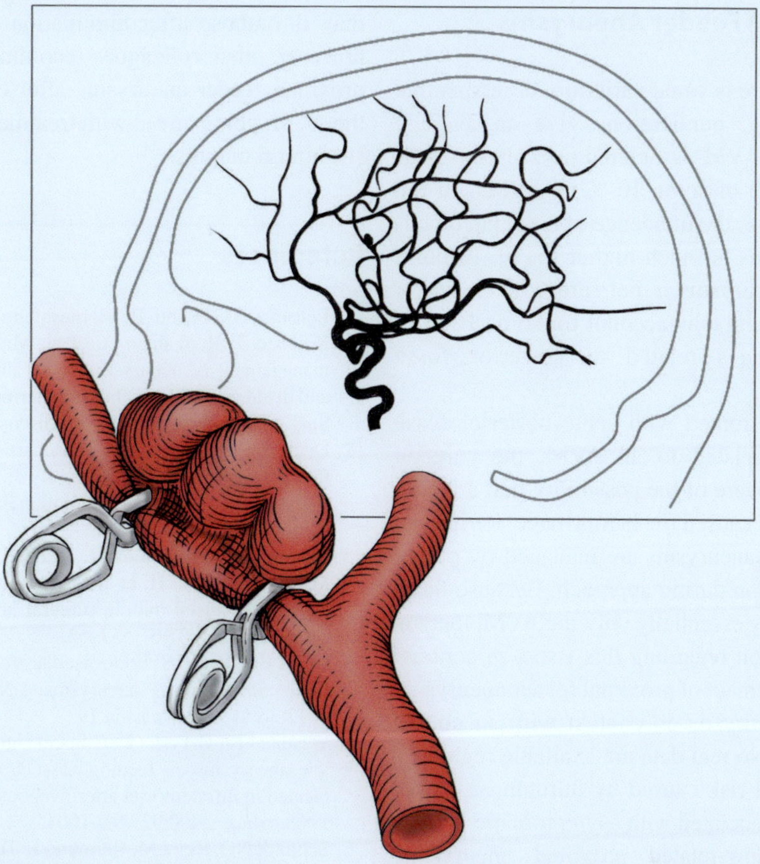

Fig. 11.2 A probably infectious peripheral aneurysm of a frontal middle cerebral artery (MCA) branch, treated by trapping and excision

11.3 AVM Feeder Aneurysms

Although there is some variation in perspective and reporting, publications give an average incidence of AVM-associated proximal or pedicle aneurysm of some 10 % of AVMs. In the posterior fossa, the incidence of associated pedicle aneurysms is much higher [5, 6]. Rupture of feeder aneurysms is not rare with posterior fossa AVMs and may account for some 10 % of all hemorrhages related to posterior fossa AVMs.

When confronted with acute posterior fossa hemorrhage related to an AVM, the surgeon needs to be aware of the possibility that a feeder aneurysm has caused the hemorrhage. Peripheral AVM-related aneurysms are managed by parent artery occlusion during approach. Because these arteries supply essentially only the AVM, there is little discussion regarding this issue, in contrast to the management of proximal feeder aneurysms or feeder aneurysms in context with an unruptured AVM. No real data are available regarding the additional risk caused by unruptured feeder aneurysms associated with asymptomatic AVMs. Regarding flow-related proximal aneurysms, some colleagues recommend aggressive AVM treatment, including the exclusion of associated aneurysms. Given that flow-related aneurysms may thrombose after elimination of the AVM, however, other colleagues recommend watching proximal feeder aneurysms after elimination of the AVM, going ahead with treatment if they persist after 6 months.

References

1. Lehecka M, Dashti R, Hernesniemi J, Niemelä M, Koivisto T, Ronkainen A, et al. Microneurosurgical management of aneurysms at A4 and A5 segments and distal cortical branches of anterior cerebral artery. Surg Neurol. 2008;70:352–67; discussion 367.
2. Ducruet AF, Hickman ZL, Zacharia BE, Narula R, Grobelny BT, Gorski J, Connolly Jr ES. Intracranial infectious aneurysms: a comprehensive review. Neurosurg Rev. 2010;33:37–46.
3. Dashti R, Hernesniemi J, Niemelä M, Rinne J, Lehecka M, Shen H, et al. Microneurosurgical management of distal middle cerebral artery aneurysms. Surg Neurol. 2007;67:553–63.
4. Gross BA, Puri AS. Endovascular treatment of infectious intracranial aneurysms. Neurosurg Rev. 2013;36:11–9; discussion 19.
5. Westphal M, Grzyska U. Clinical significance of pedicle aneurysms on feeding vessels, especially those located in infratentorial arteriovenous malformations. J Neurosurg. 2000;92:995–1001.
6. Schmidt NO, Reitz M, Raimund F, Treszl A, Grzyska U, Westphal M, Regelsberger J. Clinical relevance of associated aneurysms with arteriovenous malformations of the posterior fossa. Acta Neurochir Suppl. 2011;112:131–5.

Quality Management 12

12.1 Concepts of Clinical Quality Management

Clinical quality management includes written definition of standard procedures, the use of checklists, and regular audits comparing results with benchmarks. The targets of quality management are safety and efficacy. Because physicians have only recently accepted the need for such processes, however, the principal ideas of safety management have been taken from other fields, such as transportation and construction.

Safety concepts adopted in medicine have been profoundly influenced by the ideas of James Reason, who hypothesized that most accidents can be traced to one or more of four levels of failure:

- Organizational influences
- Unsafe supervision
- Preconditions for unsafe acts
- The unsafe acts themselves

In this model, an organization's defenses against failure are modeled as a series of barriers. Individual weaknesses in individual parts of the system are continually varying in size and position. The system as a whole produces failures when all individual barrier weaknesses align, permitting "a trajectory of accident opportunity" in which a hazard passes through all of the holes in all of the defenses, leading to a failure [1]. In the causal sequence of human failures that leads to an accident or an error, the model includes both active failures and latent failures. The concept of active failures encompasses the unsafe acts that can be directly linked to an accident, such as pilot errors in aircraft accidents. The concept of latent failures is particularly useful in the process of aircraft accident investigation, because it encourages the study of contributory factors in the system that may have lain dormant for a long time until they finally contribute to an accident. Latent failures span the first three levels of failure in Reason's model: organizational influences, unsafe supervision, and preconditions for unsafe acts. Organizational influences encompass such things as reduced expenditures on pilot training in times of financial austerity. Unsafe supervision encompasses such things as pairing two inexperienced pilots together on a flight into known adverse weather at night. Preconditions for unsafe acts include fatigued air crew or improper communications practices.

The same analyses and models apply in the field of healthcare, and many researchers have provided descriptive summaries, anecdotes, and analyses of Reason's work in the field. For example, a latent failure could be the similar packaging of two different prescription drugs that are then stored close to each other in a pharmacy. Such a failure would be a contributory factor in the administration of the wrong drug to a patient. Such research has led to the realization that medical error can be the result of "system flaws, not character flaws," and that not only ignorance, malice, or laziness causes error.

Reason's work resulted primarily in a culture of defining and periodically reviewing clinical

H.-J. Steiger et al., *Microsurgical Brain Aneurysms: Illustrated Concepts and Cases*,
DOI 10.1007/978-3-662-45679-8_12, © Springer-Verlag Berlin Heidelberg 2015

processes. Use of surgical checklists and the idea of an anonymous critical incident reporting system (CIRS) resulted from these ideas. A CIRS is not practical in a department of neurosurgery because anonymity cannot be guaranteed, in contrast to a department of radiology or anesthesiology, for example, or in the context of multicentric registries. The use of surgical checklists became popular with the introduction and validation of the World Health Organization (WHO) checklist [2]. We have been using similar checklists for more than 20 years in order not to forget preoperative or postoperative details.

Established processes to regularly verify the safety and efficacy of clinical—and particularly invasive—procedures are now expected by patients and health organizations. Although aspects of managing aneurysms and subarachnoid hemorrhage (SAH) differ from other subspecialties, it remains debatable how far quality management should be separated from the rest of neurosurgery or remain integrated in a common frame. We have regularly analyzed complications and discussed them within a common morbidity and mortality (M&M) conference for the past two decades. While trying to study the effect of these recurring audits on clear quality indicators, we realized that the main point of these audits is teaching or communicating a culture of good clinical care. M&M conferences are typical examples of case-based teaching seminars. Therefore, issues that every neurosurgeon and neurosurgical resident should know at least to some degree should be discussed together. In contrast, the degree to which separate subspecialties such as radiosurgery or functional neurosurgery can be appropriately covered in a common frame remains open to question.

Safety of treatments always has been the primary focus of quality audits. Safety parameters are simple to define in terms of complications and rates of case morbidity and fatality. Effectiveness of treatment is usually included in the analysis, as reflected by surrogate parameters such as completeness of tumor removal or aneurysm elimination. These surrogate parameters are not evidence proved, and the relevant outcome parameters such as survival rates in patients with malignancies or quality of life in patients with unruptured aneurysms realistically cannot be considered in a quality audit.

Despite the now traditional role of regular M&M conferences within resident training programs, their effect as a tool to improve quality has remained hypothetical. In more recent years, with a greater focus on quality management, these conferences have been increasingly considered to be an audit and, therefore, an instrument to identify systemic flaws. Methods of reporting cases to be discussed, methods of analysis, classification of morbidity, and criteria for consequences to improve the processes vary widely.

Quality audits can quantify defined outcome parameters such as case morbidity and fatality rates, compare them to published benchmark values, and analyze the path of decisions that led to complications. It is much more difficult to judge the quality of surgical manipulation. Quantifying precision and time efficiency of surgical acts would require video documentation of all procedures. Furthermore, analysis would require an inordinate amount of effort and time.

12.2 The Quality Management System of the HHU Department of Neurosurgery

This section summarizes the quality management system that we use in the Department of Neurosurgery of Heinrich Heine University (HHU) Düsseldorf.

12.2.1 Internal Guidelines

Perioperative diagnostic work-ups and treatment, as well as the basic surgical procedures, are standardized by written guidelines [3]. With regard to surgical procedures, standardization is limited to the approaches and the basic procedures (e.g., ventricular drainage, ventricular shunts, and evacuation of chronic subdural hematomas) that residents perform without immediate supervision. The details of the complex parts of surgical procedures, such as the technique of removing a tumor or clipping an aneurysm, are left to the discretion of the individual staff members. The internal standards and guidelines specify all those aspects of patient care that are mainly executed by residents. The main purpose of the guidelines is to provide the residents with a framework, particularly for situations when they have to make efficient decisions during on-call duty.

12.2.2 Reporting of Morbidity and Mortality

Since the introduction of regular M&M conferences, reporting of morbidity and mortality, as well as other complications such as an unplanned surgical revision or incomplete result, has been achieved by a system of classification of the hospital course at the time of discharge. The course is classified as Verlauf (V) 1 to V4:

- V1, positive, with resolution of preoperative symptoms and signs
- V2, expected
- V3, complicated
- V4, dead

This classification appears as a plain-language summary of the hospital course in the discharge note, thus allowing for crosschecking by the staff physician signing the discharge note, as well as by the patient and the family physician. The critical code V3 includes new neurological deficits and any other complication prolonging hospital stay. These complications may include thromboembolism, surgical site infection, unrelated infection such as pneumonia or urinary tract infection, or a second, unplanned surgical procedure (e.g., for residual tumor or postoperative hemorrhage). In preparation for the regular M&M conferences, the list of V3 and V4 cases is drawn from the database. Comparison with the operating room log is done in order to crosscheck for revision procedures.

12.2.3 Classification of Morbidity and Mortality

Morbidity is classified as moderate if sequels resolve within 3 months. Complications resulting in deficits of more than 3 months' duration are classified as severe. This category also includes life-threatening complications. A final assessment of the severity of morbidity of course cannot be made at the time of discharge, but only at the time of the control visit a few months later.

Mortality is classified as related to surgery or unrelated to surgery. Typical examples of mortality unrelated to a surgical procedure are fatal head injury or intracranial hemorrhage leading to death in the hospital. Mortality in relation to surgery is subclassified in terms of causal relation or not. For example, fatal postoperative thromboembolism is considered as in relation to surgery, but the surgical procedure is not considered directly causal for the mortality.

12.2.4 Criteria for Amendments of Guidelines

The incidence of classic complications such as surgical-site infection, meningitis, postoperative hemorrhage, and cerebrospinal fluid (CSF) fistulas is monitored and compared with the data in the literature. First-time occurrence of previously unknown adverse events is thoroughly analyzed and discussed. If a similar event occurs a second time, possibilities are examined that can potentially prevent similar complications with acceptable effort and costs. For example, two cases of aneurysm rehemorrhage during angiography on the day of admission were encountered. Analysis showed that there had been a shift of referral practice after SAH, so that the patients more frequently arrived only a few hours after the initial hemorrhage. Given that other reports have confirmed that angiography within the first hours following SAH carries a risk of rehemorrhage of up to 20 %, we changed the guidelines so that in case of early arrival, angiography is delayed to at least 6 h following the initial event.

12.2.5 Overall Morbidity and Mortality Rates

The key quality indicators are calculated at the HHU Department of Neurosurgery on a monthly basis in context with the M&M conference. A cumulative analysis of some 10,000 surgical procedures between 2004 and 2009 was assembled and published in 2010 [3]. The overall spectrum of surgical procedures was dominated by emergency procedures for trauma and for hemorrhage, including procedures for ruptured aneurysms (22 %), followed by spinal procedures (19 %) and cranial tumors (17 %).

Average management morbidity was 7.1 %, where 4.4 % of complications were moderate and 2.6 % were severe. Average infection rates (included in the 7.1 % morbidity) were 1.8 %. Overall, the monthly incidence varied without a discernible annual pattern. The spectrum of complications is shown in Fig. 12.1.

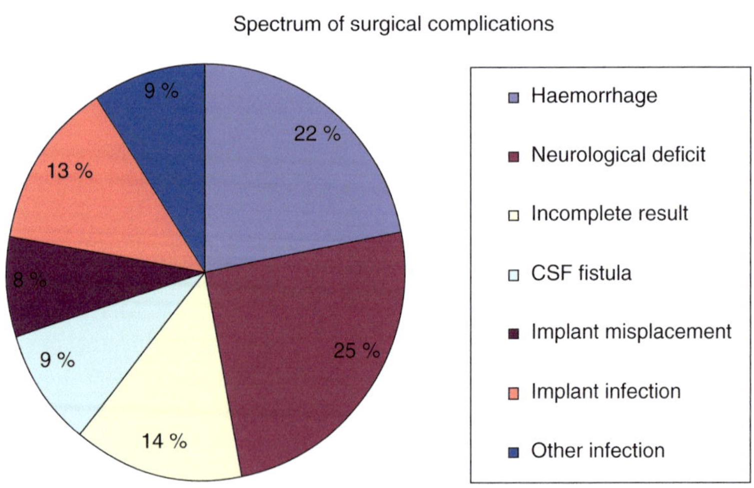

Fig. 12.1 Overall spectrum of complications in the Department of Neurosurgery of Heinrich Heine University Düsseldorf between 2004 and 2009 (Data from Steiger et al. [3])

12.2.6 Case Fatality Rates Following Aneurysmal Subarachnoid Hemorrhage

A cumulative analysis of our in-house case fatality rates following aneurysmal SAH at HHU was recently published [4]. Patients were treated for their aneurysms either by an endovascular route or microsurgically. Of the 591 consecutive patients with SAHs from ruptured cerebral aneurysms, 85 patients died within 30 days after admission. The various causes of death were classified as cerebral or noncerebral events. Case fatalities occurred after a median of 4 days following SAH. Cerebral edema as a result of initial brain damage after ictus was the predominant cause of death and occurred most often after the first day ($n=24$, 28.2 %), followed by cerebral infarction caused by delayed cerebral ischemia ($n=13$, 15.3 %; median time 9 days after SAH). Renal failure was the most predominant noncerebral cause of death ($n=6$, 7.1 %).

The in-house case fatality rates are difficult to interpret. They certainly depend to a large degree on the local setting, which determines what percentage of deaths occurs prior to hospital admission. Therefore, in-house case fatality rates have a limited importance in judging overall quality of care. The relative proportion of the leading causes of death may indicate specific problems, however. For example, fatal renal failure in six patients in this series led us to closely examine whether the frequent use of contrast-enhanced perfusion CT to monitor vasospasm might be a factor.

12.3 Management-Related Complications with Ruptured and Unruptured Aneurysms

A proper analysis of management-related complications for aneurysmal SAH remains difficult because effects of the initial injury due to hemorrhage and the effects of delayed ischemia mingle with injury due to endovascular or microsurgical therapy. Therefore, trying to extract a specific percentage from the database is an elusive goal. A comparable situation applies to situations such as traumatic brain injury, ruptured arteriovenous malformation, or traumatic spinal cord injury. It can be assumed that proper identification of complications is possible only in good-grade SAH patients and patients with unruptured aneurysms.

According to the meta-analysis of Kotowski and coworkers [5], which included 60 studies encompassing some 10,000 patients, clipping of unruptured aneurysms is associated in the reported series with an average 1.7 % mortality and 6.7 % poor outcome. Interestingly, reported morbidity rates are significantly greater in higher-quality studies. As known already from the International Study of Unruptured Intracranial Aneurysms (ISUIA), morbidity is higher with large aneurysms or posterior circulation aneurysms and in elderly patients [6]. The authors comment that the available data on surgical outcome were of poor quality, particularly with regard to minor morbidity.

References

1. Reason JT. Human error. Cambridge: Cambridge University Press; 1990.
2. Haynes AB, Weiser TG, Berry WR, Lipsitz SR, Breizat AH, Dellinger EP, et al.; Safe Surgery Saves Lives Study Group. A surgical safety checklist to reduce morbidity and mortality in a global population. N Engl J Med. 2009;360:491–9.
3. Steiger HJ, Stummer W, Hänggi D. Can systematic analysis of morbidity and mortality reduce complication rates in neurosurgery? Acta Neurochir (Wien). 2010;152:2013–9.
4. Beseoglu K, Holtkamp K, Steiger HJ, Hänggi D. Fatal aneurysmal subarachnoid haemorrhage: causes of 30-day in-hospital case fatalities in a large single-centre historical patient cohort. Clin Neurol Neurosurg. 2013;115:77–81.
5. Kotowski M, Naggara O, Darsaut TE, Nolet S, Gevry G, Kouznetsov E, Raymond J. Safety and occlusion rates of surgical treatment of unruptured intracranial aneurysms: a systematic review and meta-analysis of the literature from 1990 to 2011. J Neurol Neurosurg Psychiatry. 2013;84:42–8.
6. Wiebers DO, Whisnant JP, Huston J 3rd, Meissner I, Brown RD Jr, Piepgras DG, et al.; International Study of Unruptured Intracranial Aneurysms Investigators. Unruptured intracranial aneurysms: natural history, clinical outcome, and risks of surgical and endovascular treatment. Lancet. 2003;362:103–10.

Index

H.-J. Steiger et al., *Microsurgical Brain Aneurysms: Illustrated Concepts and Cases*, DOI 10.1007/978-3-662-45679-8, © Springer-Verlag Berlin Heidelberg 2015

MIX
Papier aus verantwortungsvollen Quellen
Paper from responsible sources
FSC® C105338

If you have any concerns about our products,
you can contact us on
ProductSafety@springernature.com

In case Publisher is established outside the EU,
the EU authorized representative is:
Springer Nature Customer Service Center GmbH
Europaplatz 3, 69115 Heidelberg, Germany

Printed by Libri Plureos GmbH
in Hamburg, Germany